YOGA FOR FLEXIBILITY

YOGA FOR FLEXIBILITY

Poses and Practices for Improving Full-Body Mobility over Time

Adriana Lee

**ROCKRIDGE
PRESS**

As of press time, the URLs in this book link or refer to existing websites on the internet. Rockridge Press is not responsible for the outdated, inaccurate, or incomplete content available on these sites.

Copyright © 2022 by Rockridge Press

First Rockridge Press trade paperback edition 2022

Rockridge Press and the Rockridge Press logo are trademarks or registered trademarks of Callisto Media Inc. and/or its affiliates in the United States and other countries and may not be used without written permission.

For general information on our other products and services, please contact our Customer Care Department within the United States at (866) 744-2665, or outside the United States at (510) 253-0500.

Some of the illustrations originally appeared, in different form, in *Pelvic Floor Yoga for Women*.

Paperback ISBN: 978-1-68539-039-6 | eBook ISBN: 978-1-68539-369-4

Manufactured in the United States of America

Interior and Cover Designer: Chiaka John
Art Producer: Melissa Malinowsky
Editor: Rachelle Cihonski
Production Editor: Emily Sheehan
Production Manager: Holly Haydash

Illustrations by Collaborate Agency; All other illustrations used under license from Shutterstock.com
Author photo courtesy of Kayla Bowen

10 9 8 7 6 5 4 3 2 1 0

This book is dedicated
to my family,
who push me to learn more about
the things that spark my curiosity.
But especially to my mother, Lourdes,
whose chronic pain pushed my curiosity
toward using yoga to feel better.

CONTENTS

INTRODUCTION

My interest in flexibility began when I started teaching yoga. My genetics gave me flexibility—my mother was a dancer, like my great-aunt before her. I didn't inherit their rhythm, but I got their natural flexibility, so I took for granted what my young body could do with ease. Once I started working with people of all ages, body types, and genetics with a variety of injuries, I realized the importance of working on flexibility.

While teaching clients privately, I met people who'd lost mobility. Some had encountered limited mobility after injuries, while others had lost it after years of decreased movement. I quickly learned that most people sit or stand for long hours without stretching, and their bodies tell the story through injury and pain. A surgeon who sat on planes for hours at a time and then stood for extended periods in surgery taught me that sitting with his legs fully extended was nearly impossible because of tight hamstrings. Touching his toes seemed impossible before flexibility work. A CEO in the tech industry with rounded shoulders and neck pain showed me how a few hours of yoga per week reduced pain and improved posture. An NFL player recovering from surgery taught me that the simplest stretches were often the ones they needed most. Everybody I worked with illustrated that using yoga to increase flexibility improved their quality of life and got them out of pain.

Flexibility isn't just for dancers, yogis, or contortionists. Flexibility helps everyone with overall wellness. As your mobility improves, you may find you're sleeping better, moving through your day with more ease and less pain, and standing taller with more strength and better balance. Perhaps you've come to this book to retain mobility while aging or to rebuild muscles after an injury. A yoga practice focused on flexibility helps in healing and in regaining and retaining strength. Developing flexibility will give you better quality of life.

I have provided step-by-step instructions for forty yoga poses plus sixteen sequences to string the poses together and flexibility plans. The sequences and flexibility plans are designed to meet you where you are. Remember: Flexibility is a journey, not a destination. There's no rush to get to any goal here. Your body may take more or less time to become more flexible—and that's okay! Continue to practice yoga for flexibility and see where your body can take you.

In this book, you'll learn how to assess your body's changing needs and adjust the poses and sequences based on that information. Work through the sequences and flexibility plans at your own pace. Consider every pose a suggestion as you move within a pain-free range of motion and use the modifications to make each pose accessible to your body. Keep in mind that while the poses or sequences in this book may include "pain relief" in the description, this book is not a substitute for professional medical care, and you should always consult your doctor before beginning any new physical practice or exercise regimen.

You'll find within all the tools you'll need to develop a regular yoga practice for better overall health. Follow the detailed instructions to feel confident getting into each pose. Add the unique sequences to your daily routine, as well as the flexibility plans, to help you achieve your flexibility goals. Whether you want to touch your toes, improve your posture, or simply feel better in your body, my hope is that this book will support you on your journey.

HOW TO USE THIS BOOK

The following chapters contain yoga poses you can do regularly to improve your flexibility, and sequences that put the poses together for flexibility training.

Follow the instructions to safely enter and exit each pose. Familiarize yourself with the poses before trying out the sequences. Some poses require warming up to prepare your body. Read the instructions and modifications before attempting any pose.

The poses fall into these categories:

- Warm-up
- Cooldown
- Backbend

- Forward bend
- Twist
- Inversion

The pose descriptions provide everything you need to know: detailed instructions, how long you should try to stay in the pose, what props you may need for support, safety precautions to prevent injuries, and pose benefits. An illustration of each pose is included as a visual aid.

Chapters 2, 3, and 4 include the poses you'll need for the sequences in chapter 5 and the flexibility plans in chapter 1. In chapter 2, you'll find basic poses, chapter 3 includes deeper stretches, and chapter 4 covers poses for pain relief.

Once you've familiarized yourself with all forty poses, you'll be ready to string them together into the sequences in chapter 5. Each sequence has a clear goal, like looser hamstrings or reduced lower-back pain. Work within your own pain-free range of motion—as a rule, each pose should be comfortable and soothing. If you experience pain, modify as suggested or try a different pose.

Consider today Point A. No matter where you are, what your experience is, or how you're feeling, this book will take you down the path to Point B—a place where your body has less pain and stress and you're on your way to living a healthy lifestyle with improved mobility.

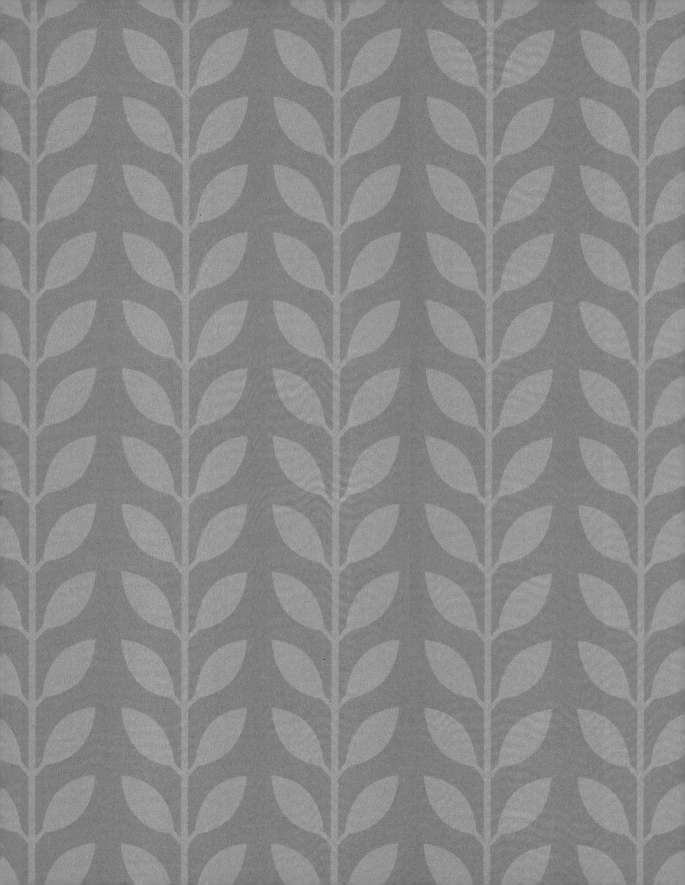

CHAPTER 1

HOW YOGA IMPROVES FLEXIBILITY

Here we'll cover basic information about flexibility, yoga, and what you'll need before you begin. You'll learn terms and definitions and dos and don'ts to keep you safe as you embark on your flexibility journey. Look for flexibility plans at the end of this chapter to help you reach your goals, from touching your toes to improving your posture and everything in between.

Benefits of Flexibility

Flexibility is about more than just touching your toes. By definition, flexibility is the quality of bending easily without breaking. Like the branches of a willow tree, your body ideally should be able to move without pain. Tight muscles can inhibit your joints from moving through their full range of motion.

Stretching regularly before or after exercise or as part of your yoga practice will lead to better flexibility. Having a higher level of flexibility will improve your ability to do daily activities, like getting to the floor and back up or walking up and down stairs. It also enables your muscles to work more effectively, which in turn will improve your athletic performance in everything from running to weight training and decrease your risk of getting injured.

Physical Strength

Rigid muscles become shortened and weak and can't fully extend. If you sit at a desk all day, your hip flexors and hamstrings stay locked in a contracted position. Then when you go to use them, for example, to walk up stairs or play tennis, the sudden strain could lead to injury.

Stretching lengthens your muscles so you can move through a full range of motion in your joints. When doing strength-building activities, like lifting weights, a full range of motion makes the exercise more effective. Strength-building also creates tiny tears in the muscles. As you stretch, your blood flow increases to the muscles and joints, delivering oxygen and nutrients, which your muscles need to heal and grow.

Increased Mobility

Mobility is the ability to move. Tight, shortened muscles inhibit a joint's full range of motion. For example, a shoulder injury can lead to restricted mobility, impairing your ability to reach for a glass on a high shelf.

Flexible muscles allow for better mobility, which becomes especially important as you age. If you don't move it, you lose it! Committing to working on your flexibility helps you maintain mobility and possibly regain some mobility you've lost over time.

Improved Posture

Posture is how you hold your body while sitting or standing. Over time, bad posture affects your health, causing headaches, pain, and even spinal injuries. Good posture promotes better digestion, better breathing, better balance, and even improved mental health.

Sitting or standing with slumped or rounded shoulders contracts the chest muscles, which causes these muscles to become "locked short," making it more difficult to stand tall. Slumped posture also holds the upper-back muscles in a stretched, or "locked long" position, making them weak. Working on flexibility, especially stretching shortened chest muscles, can help improve your posture.

Flexibility and Yoga

Practicing yoga over time has been proven to increase flexibility and balance. A typical yoga practice includes yoga postures, called asanas, that stretch and strengthen the body. Transitioning through these postures activates muscles and builds core strength, balance, and flexibility.

Most poses are held for several deep breaths, while some are passed through, and others may be held for several minutes. As you move through the sequences in chapter 5, take deep breaths to encourage your body to relax into the poses to give your body time to feel the benefits.

Resolving Muscle Tension and Pain Relief

Some muscle pain and chronic issues develop from an inactive lifestyle. Only one in four adults gets enough exercise, according to the Centers for Disease Control and Prevention (CDC). Muscle rigidity can also be triggered by stress.

Practicing yoga helps you gain flexibility and reduces stress, strengthens your mind-body connection, and helps slow down the aging process. The goal is to use yoga for your body's necessary movement and to help reduce stress to improve flexibility.

Developing a consistent yoga practice improves flexibility, helps decrease lower-back pain, and improves posture. In turn, these benefits lessen back and neck pain, reduce inflammation, and promote an overall sense of well-being. The gentle stretches and mindful breathing done in a yoga practice also help reduce the perception of pain, making pain easier to manage.

Mindset for Physical and Mental Growth and Healing

As you stretch, here are some tips to elevate your mindset for overall healing and vitality.

Slow down. When your mind is racing, take a moment to orient yourself. To return to the present moment, notice three things in your surroundings.

Get grounded. Feel your feet on the floor. Note the surface you're on and relax into the support.

Get centered. Feel the center of your body. Breathe into your belly, and as you exhale, hug your belly in toward your spine.

Take deep breaths. Do this on and off your yoga mat.

Flexibility 101

I've included the following list of some terms and their definitions to help demystify potentially unfamiliar terminology regarding flexibility.

- **Active isolated stretching:** Stretching that engages the opposite (antagonist) muscle to stretch the isolated muscle—held for two seconds and repeated 8 to 10 times—as in Half Split Pose (page 55).

- **Antagonistic muscle pairs:** A pair of muscles that causes or inhibits movement, like the biceps and the triceps. While the agonist muscle contracts, the antagonist muscle relaxes. For example, engaging the quads in Half Split Pose (page 55) utilizes antagonistic muscle pairs (the hamstrings).

- **Backbend:** Spinal extension—increasing the angle between the vertebrae of the spine, as in Camel Pose (page 71).

- **Cooldown:** Gentler exercises or poses that help the body return to a resting state, as in Pigeon Pose (page 69).

- **Dynamic stretching:** Stretching by actively moving the muscles through their full range of motion, such as moving back and forth from Low Lunge (page 35) and Half Split Pose (page 55) or by moving through Cat-Cow (page 33).

- **External rotation:** Movement of a joint away from the midline of the body like the external rotation of the shoulder in the top arm in Cow Face Pose (page 41).

- **Forward bend:** Spinal flexion—decreasing the angle between the vertebrae of the spine, as in Head-to-Knee Pose (page 43).

- **Hypermobility:** Aka hyper-flexibility, this condition allows a person to have an unusually high range of motion in their joints.

- **Internal rotation:** Movement of a joint toward the midline of the body like the internal rotation of the shoulder in the bottom arm as well as the legs in Cow Face Pose (page 41).

- **Inversion:** Any pose that brings your hips above your heart, as in Downward-Facing Dog (page 31).

- **Joint:** Where two or more bones meet, often to allow for movement.

- **Passive stretching:** Not engaging the muscles in a relaxed period of stretching. Puppy Pose (page 75), Child's Pose (page 87), and Legs Up the Wall Pose (page 103) are a few examples of this.

- **PNF stretching:** Proprioceptive Neuromuscular Facilitation (PNF), a stretching method that involves contracting (engaging) the muscle being stretched. Try this in Pigeon Pose (page 69) by pressing your outer ankle and knee into the ground to engage the outer hip muscles.

- **Range of motion:** The movement potential of a joint. A knee injury may inhibit range of motion, or how far the joint can flex or extend.

- **Reciprocal inhibition:** A process in which one muscle contracts and nerves send signals to its opposing muscle to relax. This utilizes antagonistic muscle. Try this in Head-to-Knee Pose (page 43) by engaging your quadriceps (front of your thighs) as you stretch your hamstrings (back of your thighs).

- **Sequence:** A series of yoga poses transitioned through in a particular order.

- **Static stretching:** A stretch that is held without movement, usually about 30 seconds, such as Triangle Pose (page 65).

- **Twist:** Rotation of the upper trunk, as in Half Lord of the Fishes (page 85).

- **Warm-up:** Prepares your muscles for more strenuous activity. Cat-Cow (page 33) prepares the body for poses of greater intensity.

Building a Flexible Yoga Practice

Anyone can start a yoga practice, no matter their skill or ability level. You don't need to be naturally flexible, invest in equipment, or be able to do advanced yoga postures to benefit from a yoga practice and feel better in your body.

Here you'll learn yoga practice basics to help you improve your flexibility, posture, and range of motion for better flexibility over time.

Warm-up

A warm-up prepares your body for more intense activity. The warm-up section of a sequence increases your body's core temperature, possibly to the point of a light sweat.

It's important to warm up before doing more intense yoga poses because it makes your muscles more supple for more intense and complex poses. Incorporate basic warm-ups at the beginning of every yoga session. The Morning Mobility Sun Salutation on page 108 is perfect for this.

Warm-ups can also serve as stand-alone sessions for those who are testing the waters and taking their yoga journey one day at a time.

Alignment and Proprioception

"Alignment" is a word used in yoga almost as much as "breath," but what does it mean?

Alignment means positioning your body properly in a pose to protect your joints and help you get the most out of your body. This often involves joint stacking; for example, stacking your knee over your ankle. Alignment guidelines are given from the ground up, in the same way you'd build a house, to create a stable foundation for the rest of the pose. For beginner yogis, it takes time to learn proper alignment. This is where proprioception comes into play.

Proprioception refers to the awareness of where your body is in space. You need proprioception to raise a spoon to your mouth or to step off a curb. Practicing yoga improves proprioception. The more awareness you put into practicing body alignment, the more aware you become of how your body feels in a pose. You can develop this skill by using a mirror to check your alignment or taking a video of yourself in a pose to see if your alignment looks the way it feels.

Breathing

Mindful breathing is one of the core tenets of yoga. Breath is to yoga what yeast is to baking bread. Without it, the practice is flat.

Deep, intentional breathing keeps you in the present moment and keeps you safe. It also tells your nervous system you're safe.

When your nervous system believes you're in danger, such as when you stretch your hamstrings beyond what they're used to, your brain sends signals to the muscle to contract, stopping you from stretching any further. Deep breathing turns on the parasympathetic nervous system, the "rest, digest, and heal" part, which signals to the body that you're safe, allowing you to stretch deeper.

Activation

Muscle activation helps you get more out of a pose. This helps you lift out of your joints. When sitting in a chair, you can slump and fully relax or engage your core to sit tall. You also feel this in Triangle Pose (page 65) by lifting your kneecaps to engage your quadriceps at the fronts of your thighs.

In the terminology section of this chapter (see page 4), "reciprocal inhibition" describes contracting an agonist muscle to relax the antagonist muscle. In Triangle Pose, this helps you effectively stretch your hamstrings.

You'll get as much out of yoga as you put in. To reap more benefits from your practice, activate your muscles during seemingly stagnant poses.

Cooldown

Cooling down after a yoga practice helps your heart rate return to normal and brings your body temperature back down. Your muscles are still warm from your practice and able to stretch more effectively, improving flexibility. Stretching during your cooldown helps reduce the buildup of lactic acid, so you won't feel as sore the next day.

It's highly recommended to cool down after any yoga session. Use Savasana, or Corpse Pose (page 51), at the end of every yoga session. This pose is a yoga staple, providing a clear ending to your practice and a transition back to your day.

FORMING A HABIT

It took years for your body to lose flexibility. Sporadic yoga won't give you back the flexibility you lost. But the habit of a consistent practice will. Here are some tips to make a habit of flexibility-focused yoga to help you see the benefits more quickly.

* Make the Morning Mobility Sun Salutation (page 108) a part of your daily ritual. Do a few while your coffee brews.

* Hit your local studio, rec center, or gym once a week for a yoga class.

* Do Legs Up the Wall Pose (page 103) for 15 minutes before bed each night.

* Incorporate a few seated poses during your work breaks, like Cow Face Pose (page 41).

* Before you get out of bed each morning, spend a few minutes in Banana Pose (page 95).

No matter your current mobility level or experience with yoga, by adding a few of these practices, you'll begin to see your flexibility improve.

What You Need to Get Started

While you don't need much to start a yoga practice, the following are a few essentials to build flexibility through yoga.

Time

Time is a hot commodity. You're not expected to practice an hour of yoga a day immediately. As a beginner, aim to practice one pose for five minutes daily to release tension—a simple Seated Neck Release Pose (page 83) while at work or Legs Up the Wall Pose (page 103) before bed. Once or twice a week, set aside 15 to 30 minutes to do a sequence from chapter 5 (page 105).

Once you're ready to add more, aim for 15 minutes of poses at home per day and an hour class on weekends. Over time, you'll crave more time on your mat. Work toward expanding to five one-hour practices a week.

Space

Unlike weight racks and heavy gym equipment, yoga doesn't take up much space. You'll need enough space to roll out your yoga mat with some room on all sides to move. You should be able to open your arms to the sides without hitting anything. A corner of a room is great, but the space beside your bed will do as well.

Many of the poses can be modified to be done in a chair, like Cat-Cow (page 33) or even standing poses like Warrior II (page 61). The ideal space is a quiet, warm room where you won't be disturbed.

Clothes

You don't need to purchase any new clothing to begin a yoga practice. Clothes that stretch and allow you to move freely are perfect. Loose clothing is not recommended because a loose shirt will fall over your face in inversions, like Downward-Facing Dog (page 31).

Yoga is traditionally practiced barefoot, but if you prefer to keep your feet warm, find yoga or barre socks that allow you to spread your toes and stick to the mat. Regular socks are too slippery and may make some poses unsafe. Some yogis even practice in their birthday suits. To each their own!

Yoga Accessories and Helpful Props

All you really need to get started is a yoga mat, but here are some props for support and assistance in gaining flexibility.

- **Yoga mat:** Yoga mat prices range from $5 to $150. More expensive mats last for years and can be used in any environment—even a hot yoga class.

- **Yoga blocks:** You can also use thick hardcover books.

- **Blankets:** Mexican blankets are ideal, but most cotton throw blankets or folded towels will work.

- **Yoga strap:** A belt, tie, or scarf can be used as a strap. Use soft materials for comfort.

Nice-to-Have Props

- **Bolster:** Bolsters add support and comfort. A pillow or a couch cushion can serve as a bolster. Your pillow should be 24 to 30 inches long and 8 inches in diameter. You can also use a foam roller or a stack of folded blankets or towels.

- **Chair or couch:** Some poses, like Legs Up the Wall Pose (page 103), can be done by resting your legs on a couch or a sturdy chair without wheels.

- **Eye pillow:** Eye pillows make resting poses feel extra relaxing. One that blocks out the light is great.

DOS AND DON'TS

Follow these dos and don'ts to stay safe and get the most out of your practice.

DO hold poses.
DON'T force yourself into poses or overexert.

DO warm up.
DON'T dive straight into deep stretches cold.

DO take slow, deep breaths.
DON'T hold your breath while you practice, as it may cause your body to tighten.

DO practice on an empty stomach.
DON'T practice right after a big meal. Wait at least an hour after a light meal and three hours after a heavier one.

DO drink plenty of water after your practice to rehydrate and flush out toxins.
DON'T drink alcohol immediately before or after your yoga practice. Don't drink too much water before practice, as your full bladder will be an uncomfortable distraction.

DO move slowly and mindfully.
DON'T strain or push yourself beyond your limits.

DO give your body time to recover if you feel sore or are injured.
DON'T push through an injury, as you may worsen it or reinjure yourself.

DO take modifications. If you feel tired, sick, or unstable, use props for support.
DON'T force yourself to practice when you're not feeling well.

DO use support when needed. A wall or a sturdy chair will help you balance.
DON'T endanger yourself by risking a fall.

DO listen to your body.
DON'T let your ego get in the way.

Flexibility Plans

"A goal without a plan is just a wish."

—Antoine de Saint-Exupéry

If you have specific flexibility goals for your body, these eight plans will help you achieve your goals without guesswork.

Each plan includes poses that will help you reach a particular flexibility goal, sequences to practice as you train, and ballpark estimates for how long it will take to reach your goal. Remember that everyone's bodies and backgrounds are different, so don't get discouraged if your body takes a bit longer to gain your desired results.

It's important to note that this book aims to help you reach the highest levels of *functional* mobility and flexibility. Not all skeletal and joint structures are built for contortionist-level flexibility goals, so rest assured, you won't find plans that have you putting your legs behind your head or doing the splits!

Hips and Lower Back

OPEN YOUR HIPS AND RELEASE YOUR LOWER BACK

This plan increases mobility in the hips, combats stress in the body from sitting or standing, and decreases lower-back pain.

Safety precautions: This plan is generally safe, but use caution, especially with back injuries. If you experience pain, add props until it's comfortable, or move on to the next pose.

SEQUENCE	FREQUENCY	DURATION	DAILY POSES
Lower-Back Rescue (page 114)	2x/week	1 month	Psoas Release Pose (page 97), 6 minutes Bridge Pose (page 91), 2 minutes
Sitting Rescue (page 120)	3x/week	2 months	Pigeon Pose (page 69), 6 minutes Low Lunge (page 35), 3 minutes

IMPROVE YOUR SQUATS

This is intended to unlock the hip flexors, increase hip flexion range of motion, and increase internal hip rotation for deeper squats.

Safety precautions: This plan is generally safe, but use caution, especially with knee injuries. If you experience pain, add props until it's comfortable, or move on to the next pose.

SEQUENCE	FREQUENCY	DURATION	DAILY POSES
Lower-Body Love (page 134)	2x/week	1 month	Yogi Squat (page 67), 2 minutes Downward-Facing Dog (page 31), 1 minute Happy Baby (page 47), 2 minutes
Meditative Moon Salutation (page 112)	3x/week	2 months	Cow Face Pose (page 41), 3 minutes Half Lord of the Fishes (page 85), 4 minutes

Upper Body

OPEN YOUR CHEST AND SHOULDERS

This plan increases your chest and shoulder flexibility for improved posture and less shoulder and upper-back pain.

Safety precautions: Use caution and take modifications for injuries, especially shoulder and spinal injuries. Work within a pain-free range of motion.

SEQUENCE	FREQUENCY	DURATION	DAILY POSES
Unlock Your Shoulders (page 130)	3x/week	1 month	Puppy Pose (page 75), 2 minutes Bound Locust Pose (page 81), 1 minute
Open Your Heart (page 128)	2x/week	2 months	Cow Face Pose (page 41), 3 minutes Camel Pose (page 71), 3 minutes

LOOSEN YOUR OVERHEAD REACH

This plan increases your overhead-reach mobility for less neck pain and fewer headaches, injury prevention, improved posture, and improved athletic performance.

Safety precautions: Use caution with shoulder injuries, especially if your shoulder has previously been dislocated, which makes you vulnerable to reinjury.

SEQUENCE	FREQUENCY	DURATION	DAILY POSES
Unlock Your Shoulders (page 130)	2x/week	1 month	Cow Face Pose (page 41), 3 minutes Downward-Facing Dog (page 31), 1 minute Banana Pose (page 95), 6 minutes
Invert Your World (page 132)	3x/week	2 months	Puppy Pose (page 75), 3 minutes Extended Side Angle (page 63), 3 minutes

Lower Body

LOOSEN UP YOUR LEGS

This plan is designed to increase flexibility in the major muscles of the legs to combat the effects of sitting, improve athletic performance, reduce injury risk, and decrease lower-back pain.

Safety precautions: If you sit all day, your hamstrings and hips may be especially tight, so warm up first and avoid pushing yourself into deeper stretches.

SEQUENCE	FREQUENCY	DURATION	DAILY POSES
Wake-Up Flow (page 106)	2x/week	1 month	Half Frog Pose (page 99), 4 minutes Legs Up the Wall Pose (page 103), 10 minutes
Sitting Rescue (page 120)	3x/week	2 months	Triangle Pose (page 65), 3 minutes Standing Forward Fold (page 23), 1 minute Head-to-Knee Pose (page 43), 3 minutes

TOUCH THOSE TOES

This plan will help you increase your hamstring flexibility in your journey toward touching your toes. Better hamstring flexibility improves athletic performance in sports that involve running and reduces your risk of muscle strains and sprains.

Safety precautions: Maintain a straight spine while working on forward folds, as stretching with a rounded spine may increase your risk of lower-back injury. Do not force yourself into deeper stretches.

SEQUENCE	FREQUENCY	DURATION	DAILY POSES
Lower-Body Love (page 134)	3x/week	2 months	Downward-Facing Dog (page 31), 1 minute Seated Forward Bend (page 45), 4 minutes Standing Forward Fold (page 23), 2 minutes
Fold into Peace (page 136)	3x/week	3 months	Half Split (page 55), 3 minutes Triangle Pose (page 65), 3 minutes

Spine and Neck

LOOSEN YOUR BACK AND NECK

Your spine houses your spinal cord, a column of nerves connecting your brain to the rest of your body. Spinal flexibility is crucial for an active lifestyle and optimizing your nervous system. Move your spine in all directions for better health.

Safety precautions: Stay in a pain-free range of motion when working with spinal injuries. Add support as needed to make these poses more comfortable.

SEQUENCE	FREQUENCY	DURATION	DAILY POSES
Wind-Down Sequence (page 110)	3x/week	1 month	Cat-Cow (page 33), 2 minutes Supine Twist (page 89), 4 minutes
Tech-Neck Rescue (page 118)	3x/week	2 months	Banana Pose (page 95), 4 minutes Half Lord of the Fishes (page 85), 3 minutes Cobra Pose (page 29), 2 minutes

INCREASE YOUR SPINAL ROTATION

This plan increases your spinal rotation, improving athletic performance in sports like golf, tennis, and baseball. Following this plan also helps decrease lower-back pain, increase lung capacity, and reduce injury risk.

Safety precautions: Keep a long spine as you twist. Rotate from your rib cage, not your lower back. Use caution when working with spinal injuries.

SEQUENCE	FREQUENCY	DURATION	DAILY POSES
Love Your Spine (page 126)	3x/week	1 month	Banana Pose (page 95), 4 to 6 minutes Supine Twist (page 89), 4 minutes
Wind-Down Sequence (page 110)	3x/week	2 months	Extended Side Angle (page 63), 3 minutes Half Lord of the Fishes (page 85), 4 minutes

CHAPTER 2

BASIC POSES

This chapter includes basic poses to teach you correct alignment that will prepare you for more advanced poses. These are common poses found in most yoga classes, and learning how to do them correctly sets you up for longevity in your flexibility practice. You'll find many of these poses in chapter 5 sequences (page 105), where you'll prepare your body for more challenging stretches.

The poses here include warm-ups, cooldowns, gentle backbends, and forward bends. Practice them to increase your flexibility before moving on to deeper stretches. Remember to breathe deeply and mindfully to help you on your flexibility journey.

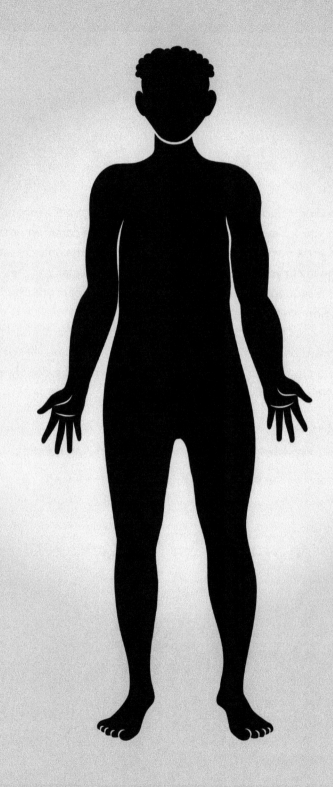

MOUNTAIN POSE
TADASANA

TIME: Stay in the pose for five deep breaths, or about one minute.
PROPS: Block or blanket
PRECAUTIONS: If balance is a challenge, stand against a wall for support.

BENEFITS:
- Improves posture and balance
- Provides a foundation for more challenging stretches and postures
- Promotes proprioception: body awareness

INSTRUCTIONS:
1. Stand with your big toes touching, heels slightly apart. For a sensitive lower back, stand with feet parallel, hip-width distance apart.

2. Engage your inner legs by hugging your ankles toward each other. Lift your kneecaps to engage the fronts of your thighs without locking your knees. Slightly externally rotate your thighs. The backs of your knees should face straight behind you.

3. Squeeze your belly upward to encourage a neutral pelvis and lift your chest. Lift each rib away from the one below it. Draw your shoulder blades toward each other to spread your collarbones and soften your shoulder blades away from your ears.

4. Relax your arms by your sides, palms facing forward. Align your ears over your shoulders with your chin parallel to the floor.

5. To exit the pose, relax to a neutral standing position.

TIP: Add a block or a rolled blanket between your thighs to encourage a neutral pelvis and strengthen your inner thighs. Experiment with different arm variations: reaching your arms overhead or placing your hands together at your heart.

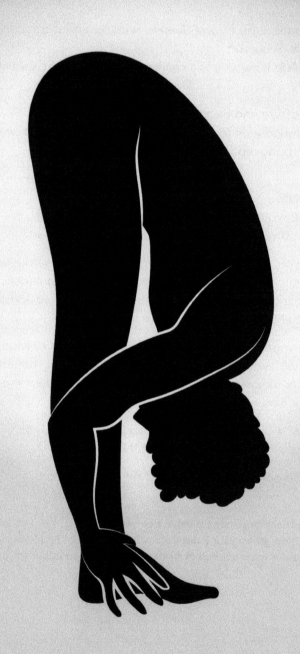

STANDING FORWARD FOLD
UTTANASANA

TIME: Stay in the pose for 5 to 10 deep breaths.

PROPS: Blocks

PRECAUTIONS: This pose is not recommended for those with eye injuries or conditions, such as glaucoma, or head injuries. Use caution with disk injuries and maintain a straight back.

BENEFITS:
- Stretches the muscles of the posterior chain (the back side of the body)
- Promotes relaxation

INSTRUCTIONS:
1. Stand with your big toes touching and heels slightly apart. For a sensitive lower back, stand with feet hip-width distance apart.

2. Hinging from your hips, bend your knees and lower your hands to the floor or onto blocks. The backs of your knees should face straight back.

3. Lengthen your spine and relax your neck. Allow the crown of your head to hang toward the floor.

4. To exit the pose, stand up.

TIP: Focus on stretching with integrity rather than touching your toes. If your hands don't easily touch the floor with a straight back, place blocks under them for support. As you become familiar with this pose, try variations. Stand with your knees bent, feet hip-width distance apart. Use your hands to grab opposite elbows and the weight of your torso to deepen the stretch.

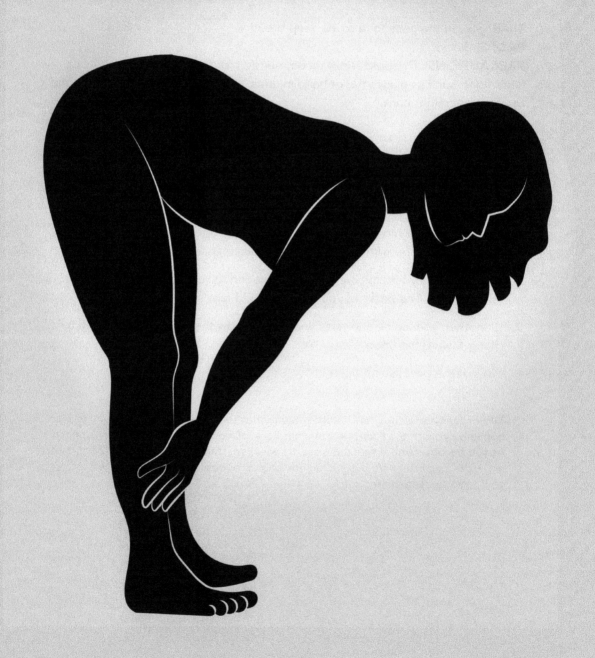

STANDING HALF FORWARD FOLD
ARDHA UTTANASANA

TIME: Stay in the pose for five deep breaths.

PROPS: Blocks

PRECAUTIONS: Those with eye and head injuries should use caution and not allow the head to drop below the heart.

BENEFITS:
• Stretches the muscles of the back side of the body
• Strengthens the core
• Improves posture

INSTRUCTIONS:

1. Begin in Standing Forward Fold (page 23).

2. Place your hands on your shins or thighs to come to a flat back.

3. Engage the fronts of your thighs by lifting your kneecaps without locking your knees. Distribute your weight evenly between the heels and balls of your feet.

4. Slightly squeeze your core muscles and flatten your back. Reach your collarbones forward and hips back. Maintain a neutral neck by looking down at the floor without collapsing your chin toward your chest.

5. To exit the pose, return to standing.

■ **TIP:** If balance is a challenge, use blocks under your hands.

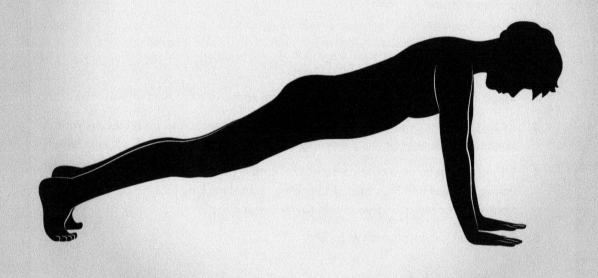

PLANK POSE
PHALAKASANA

TIME: Stay in the pose for several deep breaths, or up to one minute.

PROPS: None

PRECAUTIONS: For wrist injuries, try this pose on your forearms. Check with your doctor before attempting Plank Pose if you have shoulder injuries.

BENEFITS:
- Strengthens the shoulders, arms, and core muscles
- Improves posture
- Builds strength and stability for more advanced stretches and poses

INSTRUCTIONS:

1. Begin in a tabletop position (on all fours with knees under hips and hands under shoulders, fingers spread out, toes untucked). Walk your feet back to fully extend your legs.

2. Push the floor away and spread your shoulder blades and collarbones. Press into the balls of your feet, heels high. Engage your belly up toward your spine and lengthen your tailbone toward your heels. Engage the fronts of your thighs by lifting your kneecaps.

3. Maintain a long neck by reaching the crown of your head forward. Look down toward your mat but avoid dropping your chin toward your chest.

4. To exit the pose, lower back to your knees.

TIP: While building strength to hold Plank Pose, try modifying by lowering to your knees.

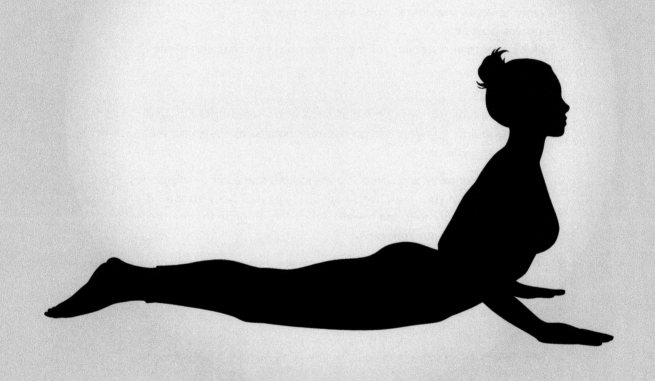

COBRA POSE
BHUJANGASANA

TIME: Stay in the pose for one breath, or longer if desired.

PROPS: Block

PRECAUTIONS: Avoid compressing your lower back. If your lower back is crunching, move out of the pose. Use caution if working with shoulder injuries.

BENEFITS:
- Strengthens the upper back and shoulders
- Stretches the chest and core
- Improves posture and counters the effects of sitting

INSTRUCTIONS:

1. Begin in Plank Pose (page 27), and then lower onto your belly.

2. Place your hands ahead of your shoulders in a goalpost shape. If your lower back feels compressed, lift one leg at a time and internally rotate it by slightly twisting the thigh toward the middle of your body; then set it back down to open your lower back.

3. Inhale and pull your ribs forward and up as if pulling yourself out of a pool, keeping your elbows bent but lifted. Roll your shoulders back and down to open your chest and press into the tops of your feet.

4. To exit the pose, exhale, and then pull your ribs forward and down.

> **TIP:** Later on, try pulling up with different hand positions, such as in a diamond shape or with your hands directly under your shoulders. It should feel like pulling up rather than pushing up from the floor. Spread the backbend evenly across your spine, without compressing your lower back, to achieve more depth. Squeeze a block between your knees or ankles to strengthen your inner legs and help keep space in your lower back.

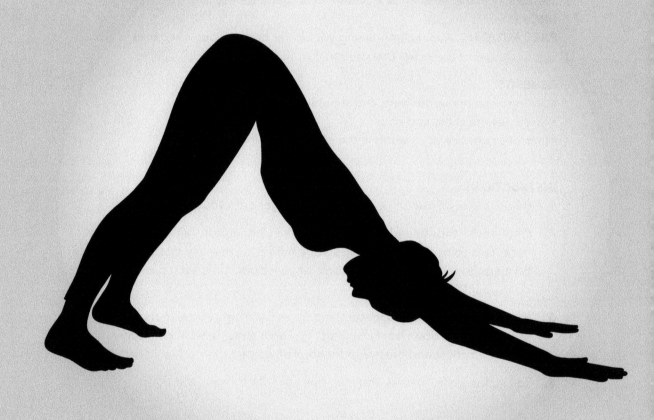

DOWNWARD-FACING DOG
ADHO MUKHA SVANASANA

TIME: Stay in the pose for three to five breaths, or longer if desired.

PROPS: Blanket

PRECAUTIONS: This pose is not recommended for those with eye or head injuries. Use caution with wrist and shoulder injuries.

BENEFITS:
- Improves balance, flexibility, and posture
- Strengthens shoulders
- Stretches the hamstrings, calves, and spine

INSTRUCTIONS:

1. Begin in tabletop (page 27). Walk back into Plank Pose (page 27), and then lift your hips up and back with bent knees.

2. Reach your hips up and back toward the ceiling, straightening your legs. If your spine rounds, keep your knees bent.

3. Spread your shoulder blades away from your spine and down toward your hips. Turn your elbows toward each other. Squeeze your inner legs from ankles to thighs and feel your inner thighs lifting toward the ceiling. Engage your core by pulling your belly in and up and relax your neck to keep in neutral (in line with your spine).

4. To exit the pose, lower back to your knees.

TIP: Beginners can experience discomfort in the hands and wrists. This discomfort typically eases after a few weeks or months of practice. Avoid hyperextending (overstretching) your elbows and knees and avoid slumping into your shoulders or pushing your chest down. Push the floor away to encourage a long spine. If your heels don't touch the floor, add a blanket under them to ground your feet.

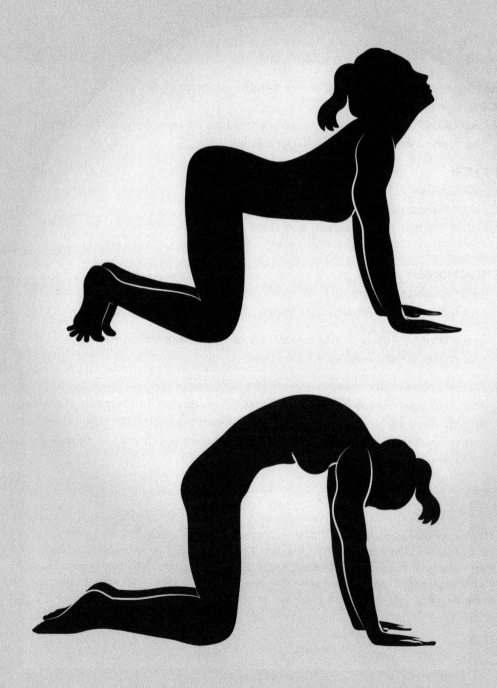

CAT-COW
MARJARYASANA-BITILASANA

TIME: Move through at least five rounds as a warm-up.

PROPS: Blocks, blanket

PRECAUTIONS: Use caution with sensitive wrists and knees.

BENEFITS:
- Warms up the spine for backbends and forward folds
- Stretches the spine, chest, and core
- Strengthens the upper back and arms
- Counteracts the effects of sitting

INSTRUCTIONS:

1. Begin in tabletop (page 27).

2. Inhale, tuck your toes and drop your spine to lower your belly toward the floor, moving into Cow Pose. Squeeze your shoulder blades together, lift your hips, and spread your collarbones wide. Lift your chin to lengthen the back of your neck in line with your spine. Squeeze your wrists toward your knees to engage your core.

3. Exhale and round your spine, untucking your toes to move into Cat Pose. Push through the palms of your hands and the tops of your feet. Pull your belly toward your spine and lengthen your tailbone toward the floor. Relax your neck, reaching the crown of your head down.

4. Repeat several rounds as you inhale and exhale to warm up the spine.

5. To exit the pose, return to tabletop.

TIPS: This pose can be done seated in a chair with your hands on your thighs. For sensitive wrists, place blocks under your forearms. Pad sensitive knees with a folded blanket.

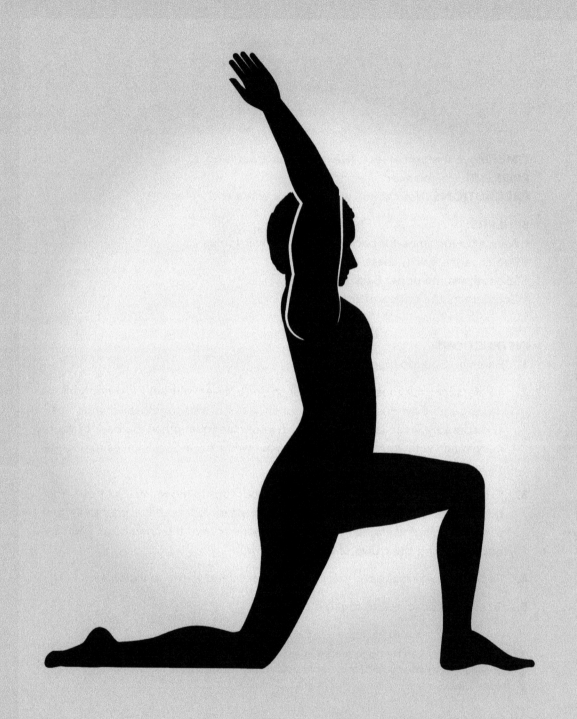

LOW LUNGE
ANJANEYASANA

TIME: Stay in the pose for about five breaths on each side.

PROPS: None

PRECAUTIONS: Check with your doctor first if you have knee injuries. For those with shoulder injuries, reach arms up to a pain-free range. For those with high blood pressure, avoid reaching arms up. Pad sensitive knees with a folded blanket.

BENEFITS:
- Stretches the hip flexors, spine, and chest
- Strengthens the legs and arms
- Improves balance and posture

INSTRUCTIONS:

1. Begin in Downward-Facing Dog (page 31).

2. Step your right foot forward between your hands. Lower your left knee onto the mat.

3. Align your right knee over your right ankle. Your right foot and left knee should be hip-width distance apart.

4. Lift your torso up so your shoulders are over your hips. Align your hip bones to face straight ahead.

5. Press your hips forward until you feel a stretch in the left hip flexors. Reach your arms up, keeping your shoulder blades relaxed. Hug your elbows in and reach up through your fingers.

6. To exit the pose, lower your hands to the mat and step back into Downward-Facing Dog. Repeat on the other side.

TIP: If stepping forward from Downward-Facing Dog is challenging, try stepping back from Standing Forward Fold (page 23). If balance is a challenge, use a wall for support, by either facing the wall or standing alongside it.

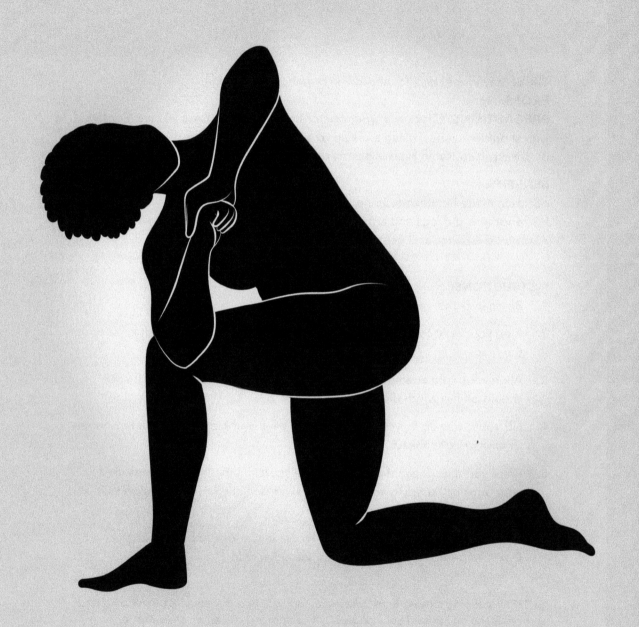

LUNGE TWIST
PARIVRTTA ANJANEYASANA

TIME: Hold the pose for about five breaths, or up to one minute, on each side.

PROPS: Blanket

PRECAUTIONS: Those with spinal injuries should use caution when twisting. Keep your belly engaged and twist only as far as it feels comfortable.

BENEFITS:
- Stretches the hip flexors, spine, and chest
- Beneficial for digestion
- Strengthens the core and spinal muscles
- Improves balance and posture

INSTRUCTIONS:

1. Begin in Low Lunge (page 35) with your left foot forward.

2. Place your hands together at your chest. Rotate your torso to the left and hook your right elbow outside your left thigh. If this feels too intense, place your right hand on the floor and reach your left arm toward the ceiling.

3. Squeeze your belly in and open your collarbones. Maintain a neutral neck, keeping it in line with your spine.

4. To exit the pose, unwind out of the twist. Repeat on the other side.

TIP: Rotate from the rib cage, not the hips. Your lower body should stay the same while you twist. Place a blanket under sensitive knees.

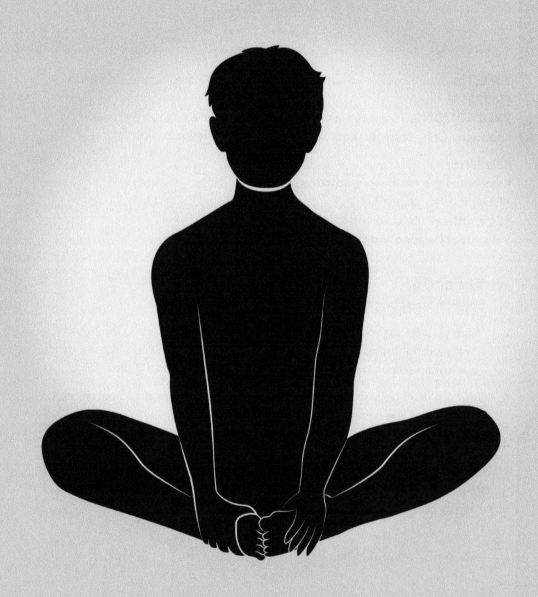

BOUND ANGLE POSE
BADDHA KONASANA

TIME: Stay in the pose for several deep breaths, or a few minutes.
PROPS: Blocks or pillows
PRECAUTIONS: Check with your doctor if you have hip or knee injuries.

BENEFITS:
• Stretches the hips, groin, inner thighs, and fronts of the thighs
• Improves posture
• Strengthens the core

INSTRUCTIONS:

1. Begin seated.

2. Place the soles of your feet together and widen your knees, letting them fall open. If your knees are higher than your hips, sit on a prop—a block or a pillow—or place props under your knees.

3. Hold your ankles and engage your core muscles to sit tall with shoulders over hips.

4. To exit the pose, place your hands outside your knees and close them like a book.

TIP: Do not force your knees down in this pose. It should feel comfortable. As you get more comfortable, try variations, like folding forward with a long spine, or try the supine variation by lying on your back and opening your knees out with blocks or pillows under them.

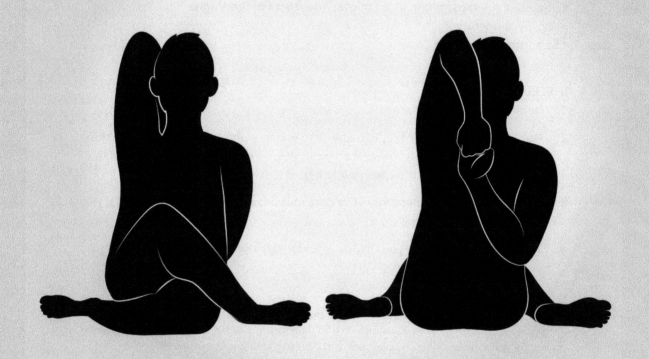

COW FACE POSE
GOMUKHASANA

TIME: Stay in the pose for several deep breaths, or up to one minute, on each side.

PROPS: Strap, block

PRECAUTIONS: Check with your doctor first if you have spondylitis or knee, hip, or shoulder injuries.

BENEFITS:
- Stretches the arms, shoulders, chest, thighs, and outer hips
- Improves internal and external rotation of the shoulders and internal rotation of the hips
- Improves posture

INSTRUCTIONS:

1. Sit with your knees bent, feet flat on the mat.

2. Grab your left ankle with your right hand and pull it to the outside of your right hip, lowering your shin to the mat.

3. Grab your right ankle with your left hand and pull it across, stacking your right knee on top of your left knee. Snuggle your ankles toward your hips. Ground your hips.

4. Reach your right hand up and pat yourself on the upper back. Reach your left hand down and behind you to clasp the fingers of your right hand. If this is difficult, use a strap, or hold onto pieces of your shirt.

5. Sit up tall. Maintain a neutral spine by engaging your front ribs down slightly to avoid arching your back.

6. Unwind by letting go of the strap or clothing and uncrossing legs. Repeat on the other side.

TIP: Keep your spine straight. Avoid leaning your head toward your elbow. If your hips are tight, sit on a block, or modify by extending your bottom leg straight.

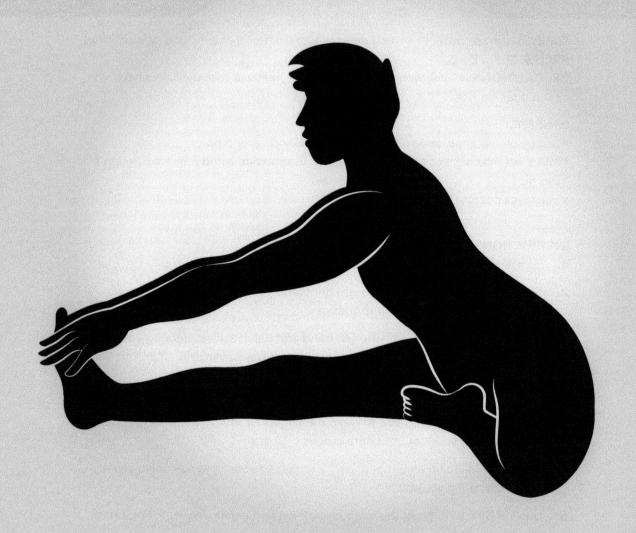

HEAD-TO-KNEE POSE
JANU SIRSASANA

TIME: Stay in the pose for five deep breaths, or longer if desired, on each side.

PROPS: Blanket, blocks, bolster or pillow

PRECAUTIONS: Maintain a long spine by reaching your chest forward rather than your hands, especially for lower-back injuries. Use caution with sciatica and follow the tip.

BENEFITS:
• Stretches the spine, legs, and hips
• Relieves lower-back tension and pain

INSTRUCTIONS:
1. Sit with your legs extended.

2. Bend your left knee and place the sole of your foot inside your right thigh.

3. Flex your right toes back toward you, aiming them toward the ceiling without letting your foot fall to either side.

4. Inhale, and sit up tall. Exhale and walk your hands forward, reaching your chest toward your toes. Hands can hold onto your leg, ankle, or foot if you can reach it comfortably.

5. To exit the pose, sit upright. Repeat on the other side.

TIP: For sciatica injuries, add a rolled blanket beneath the knee of the extended leg to keep it slightly bent. To make this more restful, set up a bolster bridge by placing two blocks on either side of the extended leg. Lay a bolster or a pillow on top of the blocks, and rest your chest on the bolster. Try utilizing reciprocal inhibition (page 5) in this pose by engaging your quadriceps, the front of your thigh, by lifting your knee-caps to encourage the hamstrings to relax and stretch.

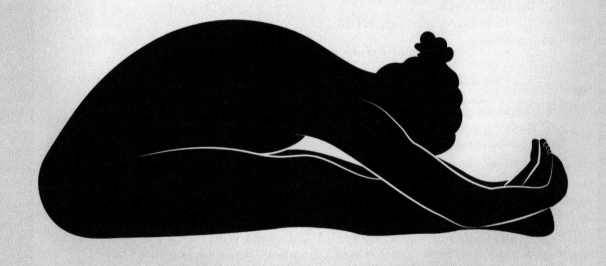

SEATED FORWARD BEND
PASCHIMOTTANASANA

TIME: Stay in the pose for several deep breaths, or up to one minute.

PROPS: Blanket or pillow, blocks, bolster

PRECAUTIONS: Maintain a long spine by reaching your chest forward, especially for lower-back injuries. Use caution with sciatica and fold with bent knees to avoid further injury.

BENEFITS:
- Stretches the back, hamstrings, and calves
- Relieves stress

INSTRUCTIONS:

1. Sit with extended legs.

2. Flex your feet, curling your toes back toward you. Toes and knees should point toward the ceiling.

3. Inhale and sit tall with hands beside your hips. Exhale and hinge from your hips. Walk your hands forward and place them on either side of your legs. Grab the outsides of your feet if possible.

4. Lengthen your spine. Guide your belly toward your thighs rather than hands toward feet.

5. To exit the pose, walk hands back and sit upright.

TIP: If sitting upright with legs extended is difficult, sit on a blanket or a pillow. To make the pose more restful, place two blocks on either side of your legs. Lay a bolster or a pillow on top of the blocks and rest your chest on the bolster.

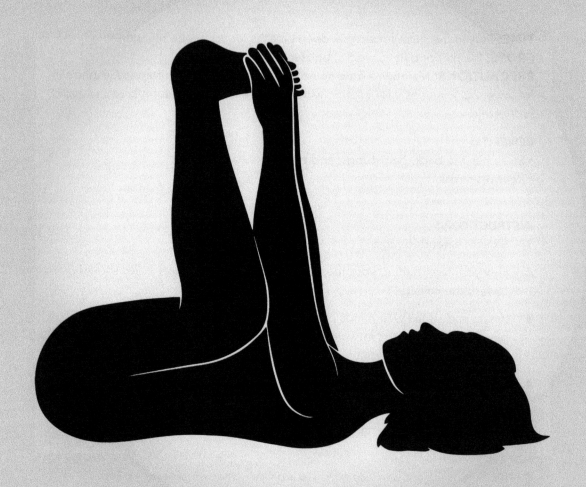

HAPPY BABY
ANANDA BALASANA

TIME: Stay in the pose for 5 to 10 deep breaths, or up to one minute.

PROPS: Towel or blanket, strap

PRECAUTIONS: Use caution with knee injuries and during pregnancy, as it's not recommended to lie flat on your back after the first trimester.

BENEFITS:
- Stretches the hips, hamstrings, inner thighs, and groin
- Relieves lower-back tension
- Relaxes the nervous system

INSTRUCTIONS:

1. Lie on your back.

2. Draw your knees into your chest and open your knees just outside your rib cage. Aim your knees toward the floor and stack your ankles over the knees, creating 90-degree angles.

3. Reach your arms between your knees and grab the outsides of your feet. If hips or neck lift, hold onto your shins or thighs.

4. To exit the pose, release your grip and lower your feet to the floor.

TIP: Keep your head on the mat. If this is difficult, place a rolled towel or blanket underneath your neck. If grabbing feet causes strain, use a strap around your feet instead. Your shoulders should stay on the floor without stress.

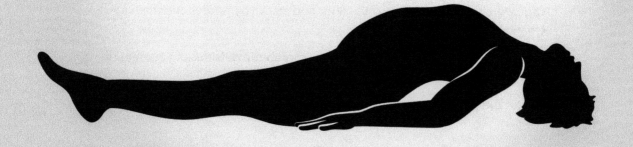

FISH POSE
MATSYASANA

TIME: Stay in the pose for several deep breaths, or up to a few minutes if desired.
PROPS: Block, bolster, or pillow
PRECAUTIONS: Use caution with neck injuries. Support your head on a block or a pillow to avoid compressing the neck. Check with your doctor first if you have high blood pressure, migraines, or lower-back injuries.

BENEFITS:
• Stretches the chest, throat, and core
• Improves posture and spinal flexibility

INSTRUCTIONS:

1. Lie on your back with legs extended.

2. Press your forearms into the mat to lift your chest. Squeeze your shoulder blades together to open the chest.

3. Relax the top of your head back onto the floor. Avoid compressing your neck. There should be no weight on your head.

4. Squeeze your legs together, activate the fronts of your thighs, and point your toes.

5. To exit the pose, release the shoulder blades and lower your torso down.

TIP: Try a restorative variation by placing a block underneath the upper back, just below the shoulder blades or between them. Add support under your head if it doesn't easily touch the floor. For a gentler variation, place a block on the mat and lay a bolster or a pillow on it to create a bolster ramp. Sit with your hips against the bolster and lie back on the ramp.

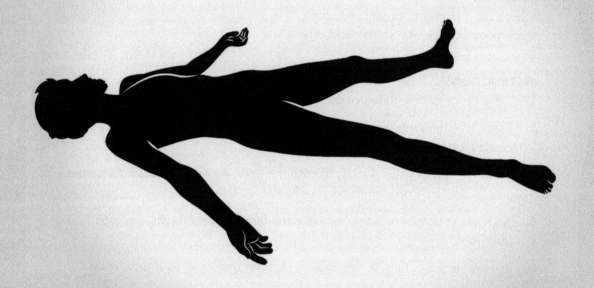

CORPSE POSE
SAVASANA

TIME: Stay in the pose for several minutes. Take one minute in Corpse Pose for every 10 minutes of practice—so six minutes in Corpse Pose after a 60-minute yoga practice.

PROPS: Bolster or blanket

PRECAUTIONS: Use caution after the first trimester of pregnancy, as it is not recommended to lie flat on your back.

BENEFITS:
• Promotes relaxation
• Decreases tension in the body, which can lead to increased flexibility
• Reduces stress, fatigue, and may help reduce headaches

INSTRUCTIONS:

1. Lie on your back, legs extended and arms at your sides.

2. Open your feet to the edges of the mat or wider. Open your arms alongside your body with palms facing up.

3. Tuck your shoulder blades under one at a time to open your chest. Tuck your tailbone under to create space for the lower back. Stay for several minutes.

4. To exit the pose, slowly roll onto one side and press up to a seated position.

TIP: This pose should feel easy and comfortable. For a sensitive lower back, bend your knees and allow them to fall in against each other, or place a bolster or a rolled blanket under your knees for support. If pregnant, lie on your left side.

CHAPTER 3

POSES FOR DEEPER STRETCHING

The deeper stretches in this chapter help increase overall flexibility and range of motion, which help reduce the risk of injury and improve athletic performance. Practicing poses like Yogi Squat (page 67) regularly may improve your squat form, while adding poses like Half Split (page 55) and Crescent Lunge (page 57) to your cooldown may help you recover faster, see faster run times, or run longer distances.

Warm up before diving into any deeper stretches and take your time entering the poses. Move with integrity. Avoid pushing further into any pose for the sake of depth. Listen to your body for what feels good instead. Some of these poses, especially the standing ones, also help build strength, which is important when working on flexibility. Take rest days if you feel sore after working on deeper stretches.

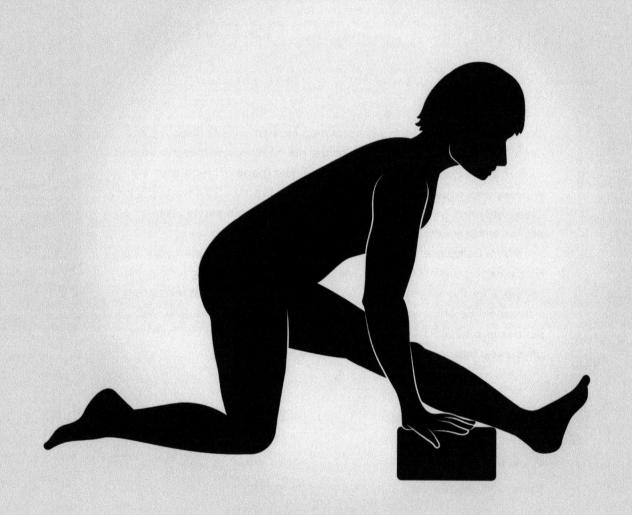

HALF SPLIT
ARDHA HANUMANASANA

TIME: Hold for five deep breaths, or about one minute, on each side.

PROPS: Blanket, blocks

PRECAUTIONS: If your knees are sensitive, pad them with a blanket. Maintain a flat back while folding, especially if you have a back injury.

BENEFITS:
• Stretches the hamstrings, hips, and calves
• Helps counteract the effects of sitting and improves posture

INSTRUCTIONS:

1. Begin in Low Lunge (page 35) with your left leg forward.

2. Lower your hands to the floor or on to blocks on either side of your left leg. Shift your hips back over your right knee and slowly straighten your left leg.

3. Fold over your left leg with a long spine. Engage the front of your left thigh by lifting your kneecap and flexing your toes back toward you.

4. To exit the pose, bend your left knee, lift your torso, and return to Low Lunge. Repeat on the other side.

TIP: Press the heel of extended leg into the ground to activate the hamstrings as you stretch. Rotate your extended leg left and right to target different muscles. If touching the floor rounds your spine, use blocks under your hands.

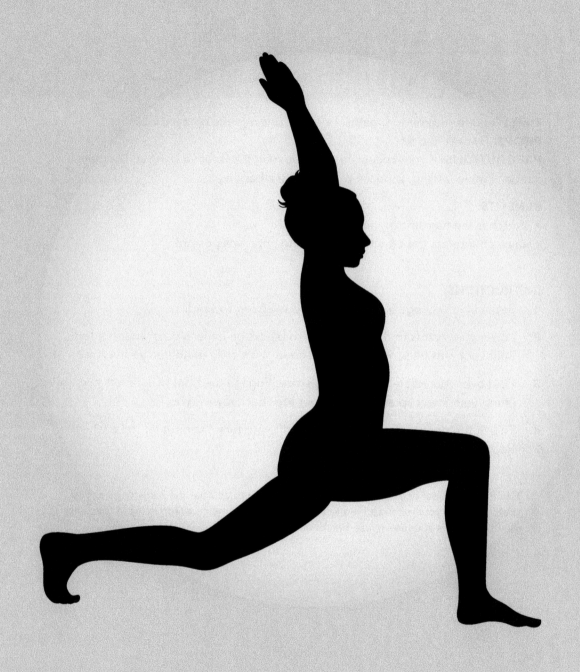

CRESCENT LUNGE
ANJANEYASANA

TIME: Hold for five deep breaths, or about one minute, on each side.

PROPS: None

PRECAUTIONS: Use caution with knee, hip, and spinal injuries. Those with shoulder injuries and high blood pressure should modify the pose by keeping the hands at the heart or on the hips.

BENEFITS:
- Strengthens the legs, glutes, arms, shoulders, and back
- Stretches the hip flexors and core
- Improves balance and posture

INSTRUCTIONS:

1. Begin in Downward-Facing Dog (page 31).

2. Step your right foot forward, just inside your right hand. Your feet should be hip-width distance apart.

3. Press into your feet and lift your torso. Adjust your stance so that your right knee stacks over your right ankle, left heel stacks over your left toes, and left knee is straight.

4. Reach your arms up with palms facing each other and shoulder blades drawn down the back. Keep your chin parallel to the floor and ears over your shoulders.

5. To exit the pose, lower your hands to the mat and step your right foot back into Downward-Facing Dog. Repeat on the other side.

TIP: Stepping the foot forward from Downward-Facing Dog takes strength and flexibility. While building the required strength and flexibility, step your front foot as far forward as you're able to, and then inch your other foot back until your front knee stacks over your front ankle.

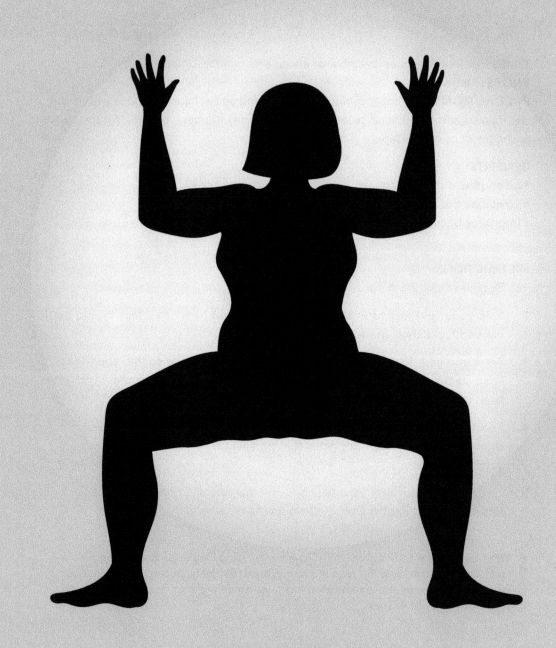

GODDESS POSE
UTKATA KONASANA

TIME: Stay in the pose for five deep breaths, or about one minute.

PROPS: None

PRECAUTIONS: Use caution and stay in a pain-free range of motion if you have knee injuries. If you have difficulty balancing, try this pose with your back against a wall for support.

BENEFITS:
- Strengthens the legs, hips, and core
- Stretches the inner thighs
- Improves balance and posture

INSTRUCTIONS:

1. Stand with your feet three to four feet apart, depending on your height, toes facing outward.

2. Bend your knees to squat. Your thighs should be parallel to the floor, but work at a depth you feel comfortable in. Track your knees over your toes rather than letting them fall in. Draw in your belly to engage your core.

3. Lift your arms into a cactus shape with elbows at the height of your shoulders and palms facing forward. With each exhale, challenge yourself by sitting another inch lower.

4. To exit the pose, relax your arms down, straighten your legs, and walk your feet back together.

TIP: Modify by sitting in a sturdy, armless chair or by standing against a wall. Activate your glutes by pressing your knees back. As your practice advances, engage your inner thigh and hamstring muscles by energetically squeezing your heels toward each other without moving them.

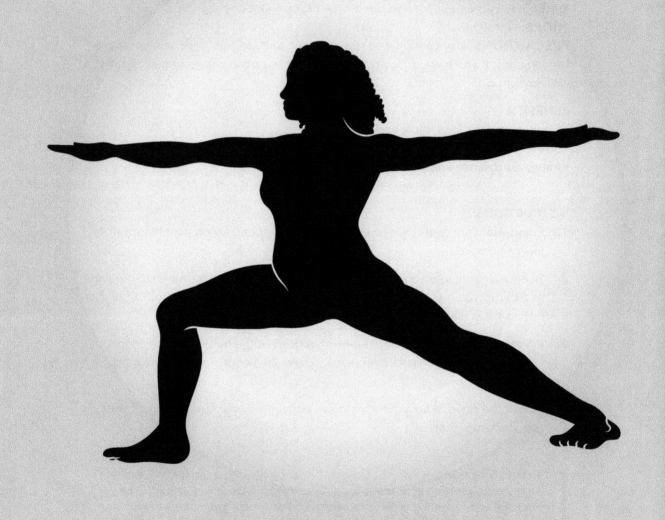

WARRIOR II
VIRABHADRASANA II

TIME: Hold the pose for five deep breaths, or longer if desired, on each side.

PROPS: Block

PRECAUTIONS: If balance is a challenge, try doing this pose with your front thigh across the seat of a sturdy armless chair, torso facing the forward, or place a block between your outer thigh and a wall. Use caution with knee injuries.

BENEFITS:
- Improves balance and posture
- Strengthens the legs, hips, and shoulders
- Stretches the legs, ankles, and chest

INSTRUCTIONS:

1. Stand with your feet wide, about the same distance apart as in Goddess Pose (page 59).

2. Turn your right toes to face the top of the mat and angle your left toes to face the top left corner of the mat.

3. Bend your right knee and push forward into it, stacking it over your ankle, with your knee tracking over your toes. Keep your left leg straight.

4. Reach your arms out straight to make a T shape at shoulder height, one forward and one back. Squeeze your shoulder blades together and down to open your chest.

5. To exit the pose, straighten your front leg and walk your feet together. Turn your feet the opposite ways to repeat on the other side.

TIP: Watch your front knee to be sure it doesn't fall inward. Press your front thigh outward so the outer knee aligns over the pinky toe side of your front foot. If you carry tension in the shoulders, face your palms up instead of down.

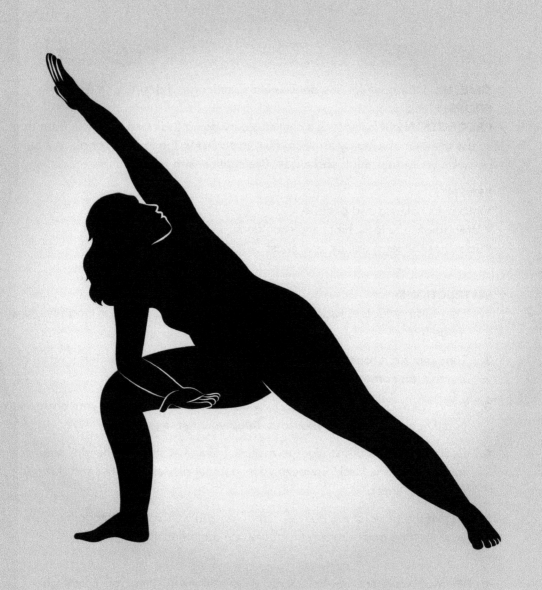

EXTENDED SIDE ANGLE
UTTHITA PARSVA KONASANA

TIME: Stay in the pose for five deep breaths, or up to two minutes, on each side.

PROPS: Block

PRECAUTIONS: Use caution with knee or back injuries. If balance is challenging, support your front thigh across the seat of a sturdy armless chair, or place a block between your front outer thigh and a wall.

BENEFITS:
- Stretches the side body, ankles, and legs
- Strengthen the core, legs, arms, and hips
- Improves balance and posture

INSTRUCTIONS:

1. Begin in Warrior II (page 61), with your right foot forward.

2. Place your right forearm across your right thigh, palm facing up. Press into your forearm and lift your rib cage away from your thigh to create space between your torso and leg rather than resting on your leg.

3. Reach your left arm overhead at an angle, creating one long line from your left outer foot up to your left fingertips. Draw your shoulder blades down away from ears and open your chest.

4. To exit the pose, lift your torso up, straighten your front leg, and walk your feet together. Repeat on the other side.

TIP: If you feel ready to deepen this pose, place your front hand on a block or on the mat outside your front foot. Your chest should face sideways or even rotate toward the ceiling slightly rather than face the floor.

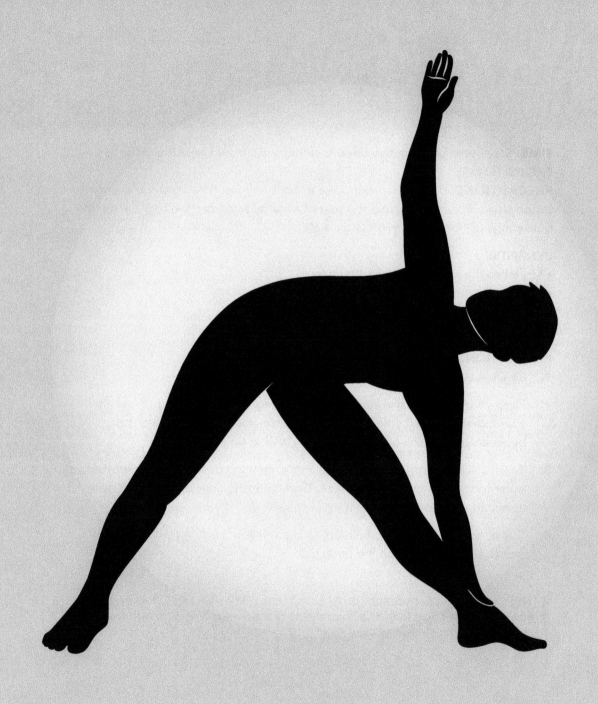

TRIANGLE POSE
UTTHITA TRIKONASANA

TIME: Stay in the pose for five deep breaths, or up to two minutes, on each side.

PROPS: Block

PRECAUTIONS: Use caution with knee, hip, and spinal injuries. Those with back injuries should modify the pose by placing a block on the front thigh and pressing the forearm into it to help maintain a long spine.

BENEFITS:
- Stretches the legs, groin, hips, and spine
- Strengthens the legs, hips, and core
- Improves balance, posture, and counters the effects of sitting

INSTRUCTIONS:
1. Start in Warrior II (page 61). Straighten your right leg and step your left foot half a step closer.

2. Shift your hips back and reach your rib cage and left arm as far forward as possible. Place your left hand on your left shin or the floor or on a block inside the left leg.

3. Reach your right arm toward the ceiling. Allow your chest to rotate out and face sideways. Squeeze your shoulder blades together to open your chest and engage the fronts of the thighs by lifting your kneecaps without locking them.

4. To exit the pose, lift your torso up and walk your feet together. Repeat on the other side.

TIP: Maintain a long spine from your tailbone to the crown of your head. Gaze at the ceiling or where your chest is facing. Avoid dropping weight into the front hand.

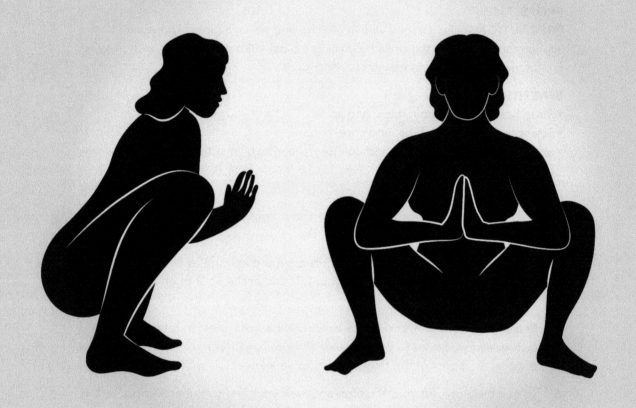

YOGI SQUAT
MALASANA

TIME: Hold for five deep breaths, or longer if desired.

PROPS: Blanket, blocks

PRECAUTIONS: Avoid this pose if you have knee injuries, and use caution with ankle, hip, and lower-back injuries. Work within a pain-free range of motion, and if you experience pain, back out of the pose slowly and carefully.

BENEFITS:
- Counters the effects of sitting and improves posture
- Improves range of motion for better squats
- Improves digestion
- Stretches the feet, ankles, groin, and hips

INSTRUCTIONS:

1. Stand with your feet hip-width distance apart or slightly wider, toes slightly turned out.

2. Bend your knees and lower your hips toward the mat, keeping your spine straight.

3. Place your hands together at your heart. Press your upper arms into your thighs and squeeze the thighs into the arms.

4. To exit the pose, stand up. If this is difficult, place your hands on the floor in front of you before standing.

TIP: If your heels lift, widen your feet or place a folded blanket under your heels to keep your weight distributed evenly across your feet. If this pose is challenging to hold, sit on a block or a stack of blocks for support.

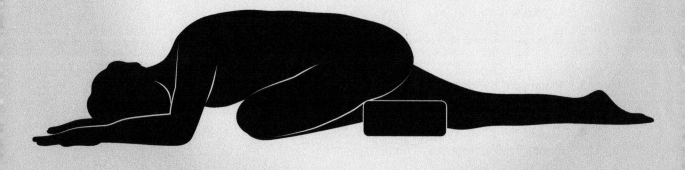

PIGEON POSE
EKA PADA RAJAKAPOTASANA

TIME: Hold the pose for five deep breaths, or up to 10 minutes, on each side.

PROPS: Block or thick book, blanket or pillow or bolster

PRECAUTIONS: If you have a knee injury or sciatica, practice Star-Shaped Pigeon (page 101) instead.

BENEFITS:
- Increases hip mobility, including external rotation of the thigh bone in the hip joint
- Stretches the outer hip, hip flexors, and lower back
- May support healthy digestion

INSTRUCTIONS:
1. Begin in tabletop (see page 27).

2. Slide your left shin forward and lower it to the floor. Place a prop underneath your left hip bone for support if it doesn't touch the ground. Reach your right leg straight back and untuck your toes to point behind with heel facing the ceiling.

3. Inhale and reach your rib cage forward. Exhale and lower your forearms to the floor. Place your forehead on the mat or a prop, or stack your hands or forearms to make a pillow for your head.

4. To exit the pose, walk your hands back under your shoulders and lift your torso. Tuck your right toes and slide your right knee forward and left knee back, returning to tabletop. If exiting the pose this way is uncomfortable, remove the prop from underneath your left hip. Lower your hip onto the floor and bend your back knee. Slide your right leg forward until you are in a seated position. Repeat on the other side.

> **TIP:** This should feel like a resting pose. Release your jaw and relax your muscles. If the pose feels too intense, add more support underneath the hip. If your sit bones don't reach the floor, sit on a block, thick book, folded blanket, pillow, or bolster. If holding the pose for an extended period, practice it with support. If your head doesn't reach the floor, place props beneath your torso.

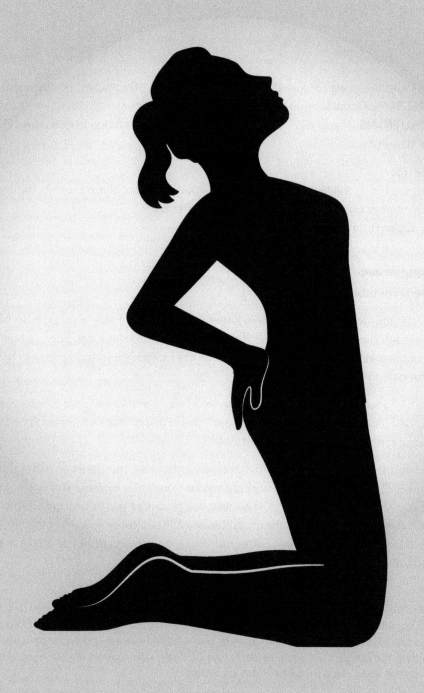

CAMEL POSE
USTRASANA

TIME: Stay in the pose for three to five deep breaths, or up to one minute.
PROPS: Blanket, block, or pillow
PRECAUTIONS: Use caution with spinal injuries. Avoid dropping your head back, as this compresses the nerves and can cause dizziness.

BENEFITS:
• Stretches the chest, shoulders, and hip flexors
• Strengthens the back muscles, backs of the legs, and glutes
• Improves posture

INSTRUCTIONS:
1. Begin on your knees with legs hip-width distance apart. Press the tops of your feet into the mat or tuck your toes under if that feels more comfortable for the knees.

2. Place your hands behind you on either side of your sacrum, the triangular bone at the base of the spine, with fingers pointing down. For sensitive wrists, make fists instead.

3. Lengthen your tailbone down and lift your rib cage up. Slowly arch your back, creating space between the vertebrae of the spine. Squeeze your shoulder blades together and down. Lengthen your neck without dropping the head back.

4. To exit the pose, lift your torso and sit back on your heels.

TIP: Place a blanket under your knees for cushioning. Squeeze a block or pillow between your thighs to strengthen your thighs. Enter the pose mindfully, focusing on lengthening the spine rather than pushing for depth. As you advance, try lowering your hands onto your heels.

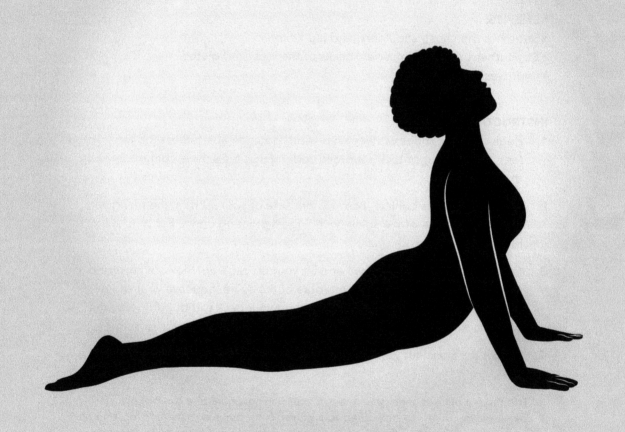

UPWARD-FACING DOG
URDHVA MUKHA SVANASANA

TIME: Hold the pose for one to five deep breaths, or up to one minute.

PROPS: Blocks

PRECAUTIONS: Use caution with shoulder and spinal injuries. For a sensitive lower back, add blocks under your hands to decrease the intensity of the back-bend. For sensitive wrists, practice on fists with your palms facing each other and thumbs on the mat, or avoid this pose if you still experience wrist pain.

BENEFITS:
• Improves posture and counters the effects of sitting
• Strengthens the back muscles, arms, and wrists
• Stretches the chest, shoulders, and core

INSTRUCTIONS:

1. Lie on your belly with feet hip-width distance apart. Slightly internally rotate your thighs to spiral the inner thighs toward the ceiling and create space in your lower back. Place your hands on the mat directly under your shoulders.

2. Push your hands into the mat to straighten your arms and lift your knees from the floor. Press the tops of your feet down to engage the fronts of your thighs and squeeze your ankles toward each other. Reach your heart forward. Lengthen the back of your neck without dropping your head back.

3. To exit the pose, lower your knees and press back into a seated position.

TIP: Shoulders sliding up to the ears is a sign you're dropping your weight into the wrists rather than actively pushing into the floor. If maintaining your legs lifted is difficult, work on Cobra Pose (page 29) to build strength.

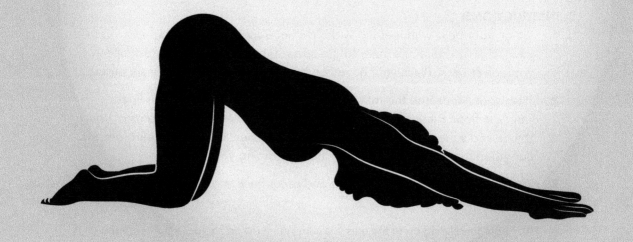

PUPPY POSE
UTTANA SHISHOSANA

TIME: Hold the pose for five deep breaths, or up to a few minutes.

PROPS: Block, blanket, or pillow

PRECAUTIONS: Avoid this pose if you have shoulder injuries. Use caution with knee, spine, or hip injuries.

BENEFITS:
- Stretches the upper back, shoulders, and spine
- Improves posture and counters the effects of sitting

INSTRUCTIONS:

1. Begin in tabletop (see page 27).

2. Walk your hands forward and lower your chest toward the floor, keeping your hips high and stacked over your knees.

3. Place your forehead on the floor or on a prop if it doesn't reach. Press into the tops of your feet and slightly pull your belly in. Press your hands firmly into the mat and keep your elbows slightly lifted, arms engaged.

4. To exit the pose, lower your hips to your heels.

TIP: Avoid letting your rib cage drop forward too much, as this compresses the lower back and takes away from the shoulder stretch. Instead, draw your front ribs in slightly. If your head doesn't reach the floor, add a block, folded blanket, or pillow under your forehead. Pad sensitive knees with a folded blanket.

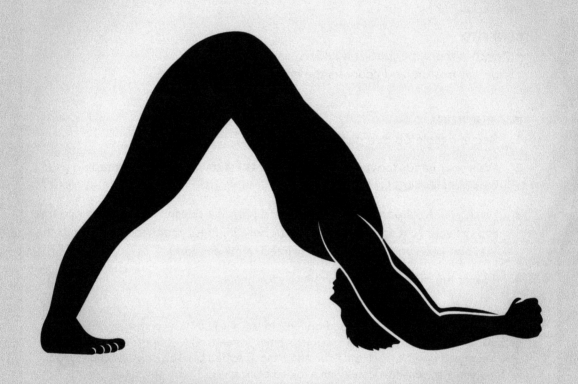

DOLPHIN POSE
ARDHA PINCHA MAYURASANA

TIME: Hold the pose for five deep breaths, or up to two minutes.
PROPS: None
PRECAUTIONS: This pose is not recommended for those with eye or head injuries or anyone who's had a recent stroke. Use caution with shoulder injuries.

BENEFITS:
• Stretches the spine, shoulders, hamstrings, calves, and ankles
• Strengthens the shoulders, and core

INSTRUCTIONS:

1. Begin in tabletop (see page 27). Lower your forearms.

2. Clasp your hands around your upper arms to determine where your elbows should be, and then straighten your forearms out into a number 11 shape or modify by interlacing your fingers.

3. Tuck your toes and lift your hips up and back, straightening your spine. Straighten your legs and press back into your heels. If your spine rounds, bend your knees. Actively push the floor away with your forearms and energetically squeeze your elbows toward each other without moving them. Let go of tension in the neck by allowing your head to hang.

4. To exit the pose, lower back to your knees.

TIP: If your elbows slide out to the sides, clasp your hands together or face your palms toward each other, which engages the biceps more and may help stabilize the pose.

CHAPTER 4

POSES FOR PAIN RELIEF

The poses in this chapter help relieve pain, reduce tension in the body, and counteract the effects of sitting. These poses move the spine in all directions and help improve overall mobility.

Practice them daily and add them to any yoga sequence, especially as cooldown poses. Be sure to breathe deeply and move slowly. These are gentler stretches that can—and should—be held for longer periods. Props are encouraged and can make these poses feel more restful.

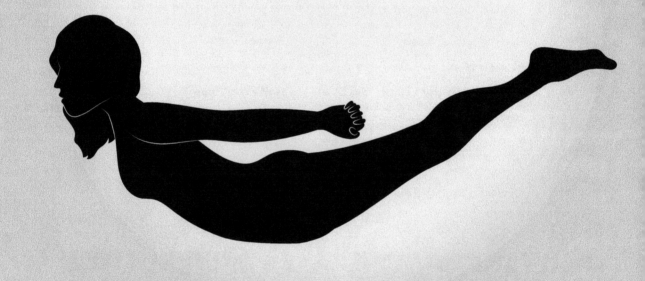

BOUND LOCUST POSE
BADDHA HASTA SALABHASANA

TIME: Hold for 5 to 10 deep breaths, or about one minute.
PROPS: Strap
PRECAUTIONS: Spread the bend across the back evenly to avoid compressing the lower back, especially if you have back injuries or sciatica. Avoid this pose while pregnant.

BENEFITS:
• Strengthens the back, abdominals, hamstrings, and glute muscles
• Stretches the chest and shoulders
• Improves posture and counters the effects of sitting
• May relieve sciatica and lower-back pain

INSTRUCTIONS:
1. Lie on your belly with feet hip-width distance apart and arms by your sides.

2. Slightly internally rotate your thighs by spiraling the inner thighs toward the ceiling. Clasp your hands together behind your back. If you can't reach, hold on to a strap.

3. Lift your chest and legs up. Keep your legs straight and squeeze your inner legs so they don't splay out wider than hip-width distance apart.

4. Lift your hands off your back and straighten your arms as much as possible while keeping the hands clasped together.

5. To exit the pose, lower onto your belly.

TIP: Avoid bending your knees. Focus on evenly distributing the backbend rather than lifting as high as you can. Keep your head in line with your spine by looking down or slightly forward.

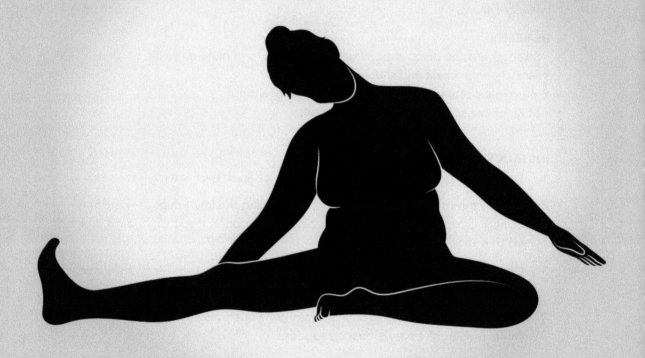

SEATED NECK RELEASE POSE

TIME: Hold for five deep breaths, or longer if desired, on each side.
PROPS: Block or blanket
PRECAUTIONS: For hamstring injuries, sit cross-legged in this pose.

BENEFITS:
• Releases tension and pain from the neck and shoulders
• May reduce headaches
• Improves posture
• Relaxes the nervous system
• Mild stretch for the hamstrings and side body

INSTRUCTIONS:
1. Begin seated. Extend your right leg out to the side and place your left foot inside your right inner thigh. If your hips are tight, sit on a block or a folded blanket.

2. Place your right hand down to the right of your right hip. Reach your left arm to the side, hovering the fingertips just above the mat.

3. Ease your right ear down toward your right shoulder. Roll your chin forward and back slightly to find the angle that feels best for your neck. Relax your shoulder blades down your back and relax your jaw.

4. To exit the pose, use your right hand to lift your head back to neutral with a relaxed neck, and return to seated. Repeat on the other side.

TIP: This pose should help release tension rather than feel like a deep neck stretch. Practice a variation of it throughout the workday while seated at your desk.

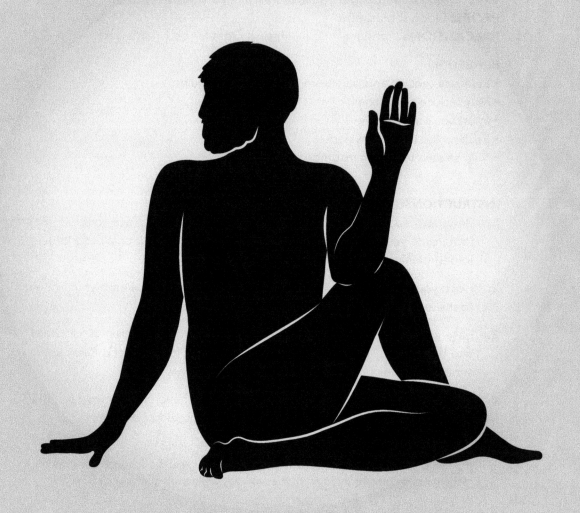

HALF LORD OF THE FISHES
ARDHA MATSYENDRASANA

TIME: Hold for five deep breaths, or longer if desired, on each side.

PROPS: None

PRECAUTIONS: If pregnant, twist the opposite way to avoid compressing the belly. Those with spinal injuries and sciatica benefit from this pose but must practice mindfully, with a focus on lengthening the spine. Do not force a deeper twist.

BENEFITS:
- Improves digestion
- May reduce lower-back and sciatica pain, and counters the effects of sitting
- Stretches the back, core, outer hips, and thighs
- Strengthens the back and core muscles
- Opens the chest, improving posture

INSTRUCTIONS:

1. Sit with your legs extended. Cross your right leg over your left, grounding your right foot outside your left thigh. Slide your left ankle toward your body to rest outside your right hip. Press down through your right foot.

2. Sit up tall, inhale, and reach your left arm toward the ceiling. As you exhale, rotate your rib cage to the right, placing your right hand or fingertips on the mat behind you, and either bring your left elbow outside your right knee or wrap your left arm around your right thigh to squeeze the thigh in and maintain a tall spine.

3. To exit the pose, unwind from the twist and uncross your legs. Repeat on the other side.

TIP: If bringing your right foot to the floor outside the thigh while bending the left leg is challenging, try extending the left leg long instead.

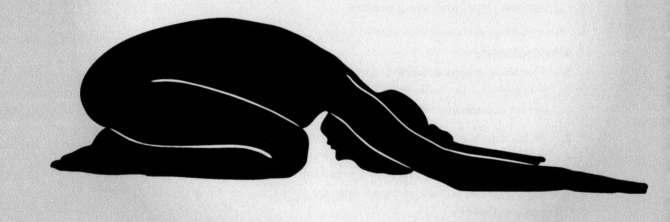

CHILD'S POSE
BALASANA

TIME: Hold for five deep breaths, or up to 10 minutes.

PROPS: Blanket, bolster, or pillow

PRECAUTIONS: Avoid this pose if you have knee injuries. For shoulder injuries, relax your arms by your sides with palms facing up. If pregnant, widen the knees to allow space for your belly.

BENEFITS:
- Stretches the lower back, hips, fronts of the thighs, and ankles
- May help reduce back pain, menstrual cramps, and hip tension
- Relaxes the nervous system

INSTRUCTIONS:
1. Begin in tabletop (see page 27). Widen your knees and bring your big toes to touch behind you.

2. Ease your hips back onto your heels and walk your hands forward. Lower your forehead to the mat and reach your arms straight out in front of you. Close your eyes and let go of tension in your shoulders, neck, and jaw.

3. To exit the pose, walk your hands back under your shoulders, straighten your arms, and walk your knees back in to return to tabletop.

> **TIP:** Add props for comfort and support. Place a rolled blanket under sensitive ankles. Add a blanket, bolster, or pillow between your calves and thighs to help with knee sensitivity and tight quadriceps. Place a bolster, pillow, or blankets under your chest and head to make this pose more restful.

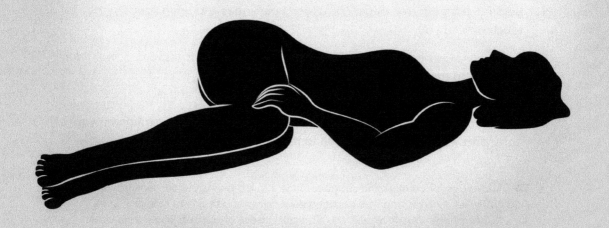

SUPINE TWIST
SUPTA MATSYENDRASANA

TIME: Hold the pose for five breaths or longer if desired, up to 10 minutes, on each side.

PROPS: Pillow, bolster, or blanket

PRECAUTIONS: Rotate from the rib cage, not the hips, to avoid stressing the sacroiliac joints (the joints on either side of the bony plate at the base of the spine) and causing instability in the joints.

BENEFITS:
- Relieves lower-back pain and menstrual cramps
- Stretches the back muscles, core, and outer hips
- Improves digestion and posture
- May be relaxing for the nervous system

INSTRUCTIONS:

1. Lie on your back. Pull your knees into your chest and roll onto your left side.

2. Stack the hips, knees, and ankles, making a 90-degree angle with your legs. Your knees should be at the height of your belly button.

3. Rest your left hand on your belly or top thigh. Twist your chest open toward the ceiling without moving the lower body. If your right shoulder blade touches the floor, open your right arm to that side. If the shoulder blade is lifted, reach your right arm overhead with palm facing down to protect the shoulder, or support it with a pillow or folded blanket.

4. To exit the pose, roll onto your back. Repeat on other side.

TIP: Face the direction that is most comfortable for your neck. Add a pillow, bolster, or folded blanket between your knees for comfort.

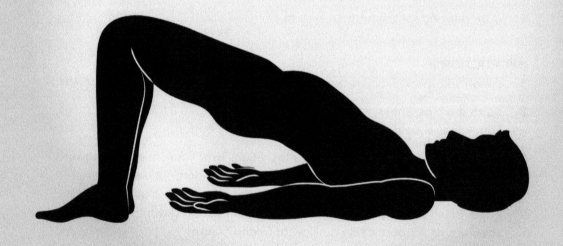

BRIDGE POSE
SETU BANDHA SARVANGASANA

TIME: Hold for five deep breaths, or longer if desired.

PROPS: Small towel, block, bolster

PRECAUTIONS: This pose is not recommended after the first trimester of pregnancy. If you have a neck injury or hernia, check with your doctor before attempting.

BENEFITS:
- Strengthens the legs and hips
- Stretches the hip flexors, abdominals, quadriceps, and chest
- Improves posture and counters the effects of sitting
- Helps relieve lower-back pain and menstrual cramps
- Improves digestion

INSTRUCTIONS:
1. Lie on your back with knees bent and feet flat on the floor, hip-width distance apart. Stack your knees over your ankles. Place your arms by your sides, palms facing up.

2. Press into your feet and slowly roll your hips up, leading with the tailbone. Push your heels down and energetically pull them back toward your shoulders without moving your feet, activating the backs of your legs. Relax your arms and avoid using your shoulders to push yourself up.

3. To exit the pose, roll your hips back down.

TIP: If your neck bothers you, try placing a small rolled towel under it. To strengthen the inner legs, squeeze a block between your ankles or thighs. For more support or to make the pose more restful, place a block or a bolster under your sacrum, the triangular bone at the base of the spine.

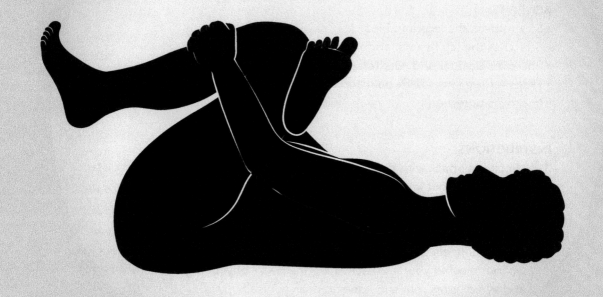

RECLINED FIGURE-FOUR POSE
SUCIRANDHRASANA

TIME: Hold for five deep breaths, or longer if desired, on each side.
PROPS: Strap or towel
PRECAUTIONS: Use caution with knee and hip injuries and recent surgeries.
Modify this pose in the second and third trimesters of pregnancy by sitting in a
chair to avoid compressing the belly.

BENEFITS:
• Stretches the outer hips and hamstrings
• Releases tension in the lower back
• May help relieve sciatica and lower-back pain

INSTRUCTIONS:
1. Lie on your back with knees bent and feet flat on the mat hip-width
   distance apart.

2. Cross your right ankle over your left thigh, making a number four shape. Flex
   your foot by pointing your toes toward the ceiling to protect the knee.

3. Pull your left knee toward your left shoulder. Reach your right hand between
   your legs and left hand outside the thigh. Grab your left thigh, shin, or clothing to pull your knee closer. Keep your hips, shoulders, and neck grounded. If
   deepening the pose causes you to lift, back out of it.

4. To exit the pose, release your leg and lower both feet back to the floor.
   Repeat on the other side.

TIP: If reaching the thigh is challenging, loop a strap or towel around your thigh to
pull the leg closer.

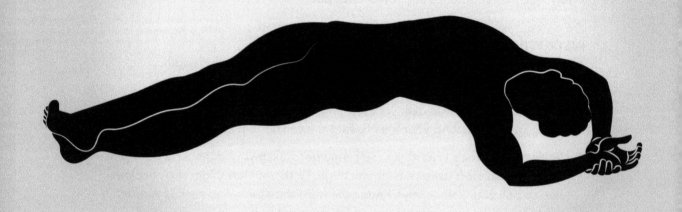

BANANA POSE
BANANASANA

TIME: Stay in the pose for 10 deep breaths, or up to several minutes, on each side.

PROPS: Blanket or pillow

PRECAUTIONS: If you experience tingling or numbness in the arms or hands, adjust the position of your arms, use a folded blanket or a pillow to elevate your arms, or place your arms by your sides.

BENEFITS:
- Stretches the muscles and connective tissues of the side body, including the rib cage, obliques, outer hips, and outer legs
- May help reduce back pain, hip tension, and knee pain
- Improves side-to-side flexion and mobility of the spine
- May help improve digestion

INSTRUCTIONS:

1. Lie on your back with legs extended.

2. Scoot your hips a few inches to the right and slide your legs to the left. Both hips should remain on the floor. Reach your arms overhead and slide them to the left, holding opposite wrists or elbows with opposite hands. Cross your right ankle over your left ankle to deepen the stretch. Shoulders should be on the floor. Breathe deeply and avoid tensing.

3. To exit the pose, uncross your ankle and slide your arms, legs, and hips back to center. Repeat on the opposite side.

TIP: You may not feel a deep stretch immediately. Wait a minute or so before adjusting to find a deeper stretch, as the sensation may take time to build.

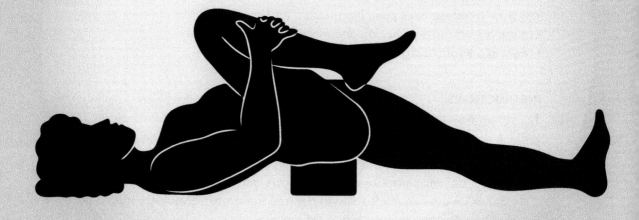

PSOAS RELEASE POSE

TIME: Hold for 2 to 10 minutes on each side.

PROPS: Block, bolster, foam roller, or blanket stack; strap

PRECAUTIONS: Work in a pain-free range of motion if you have spine or hip injuries to avoid aggravating the injury.

BENEFITS:
- Stretches the hip flexors
- Relieves lower-back tension and pain
- Improves posture and counters the effects of sitting
- Relaxes the nervous system

INSTRUCTIONS:

1. Lie on your back with knees bent and feet flat on the mat.

2. Lift your hips, as in Bridge Pose (page 91), and then slide a prop under your hips, resting upper glutes (bottom) on it.

3. Draw your right knee into your chest. Hold on to your shin or thigh or loop a strap under the thigh. Use the weight of the leg to help relax your rib cage down toward the floor.

4. Extend your left leg forward. If your heel lifts, place a block under it.

5. To exit the pose, bend your left knee and place your foot on the floor. Lower your right foot down. Lift your hips and remove the prop; then lower your hips to the floor. Repeat on the other side.

TIP: Breathe deeply and hold the pose for as long as you can, ideally five minutes or more per side.

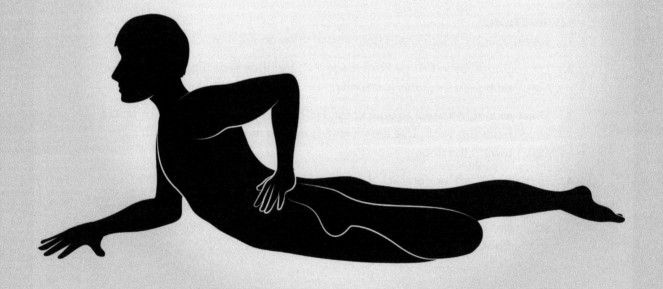

HALF FROG POSE
ARDHA BHEKASANA

TIME: Remain in the pose for five deep breaths or longer on each side.

PROPS: Strap or belt

PRECAUTIONS: Avoid this pose if you have arthritis in your knees or ankles, or if you're in the second or third trimester of pregnancy. Use caution with knee and spine injuries.

BENEFITS:
- Stretches the fronts of the thighs, hip flexors, and core
- Strengthen the back muscles
- Improves posture and counters the effects of sitting
- May reduce lower-back pain, knee pain, and hip pain

INSTRUCTIONS:

1. Lie on your belly. Rotate your thighs slightly inward and spread the tops of your toes into the floor.

2. Lift your chest and place your forearms down, stacking elbows under shoulders.

3. Turn your right hand in so your forearm is at a diagonal. Bend your left knee and use your left hand to pull your left foot toward your glutes (bottom). If flexibility allows, turn your fingers to face forward, with hand on the top of the foot, and gently press down.

4. Press both hipbones down. Using your right forearm, energetically pull your chest forward. Keep your chest lifted and spread your collarbones.

5. To exit the pose, release your leg and return your left elbow under your shoulder. Lower your chest down. Repeat on the opposite side.

■ **TIP:** If you can't quite reach your foot, loop a strap or a belt around it.

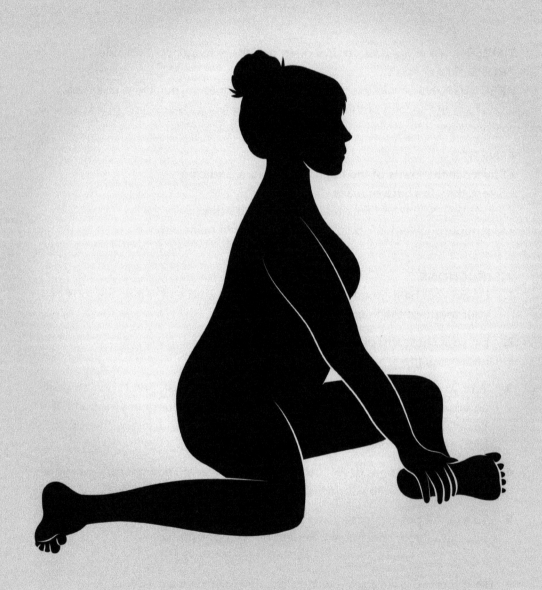

STAR-SHAPED PIGEON

TIME: Hold for five deep breaths, or one minute, per side.
PROPS: Blanket or block
PRECAUTIONS: If you experience pain, adjust the pose until it's comfortable, or exit the pose.

BENEFITS:
• May relieve sciatica and lower-back pain
• Stretches most of the muscles of the hips
• Increases internal and external rotation and overall hip mobility
• Strengthens the core and back muscles

INSTRUCTIONS:
1. Sit in a cross-legged position. Bend your left leg in front of you, forming a ninety degree angle on the floor.

2. Swing your right knee back and place it in line with your right hip, with inner knee and ankle on the floor. This forms a second 90-degree angle. If it's too much, slide your right knee forward or back until it's comfortable.

3. Press both legs down and sit with a straight spine. If your spine rounds, elevate your front hip with a folded blanket or a block. Avoid leaning to the side.

4. To exit the pose, slide your back leg forward and return to seated. Repeat on the other side.

TIP: This pose is sometimes called 90-90 because your legs form two 90-degree angles. If it's too difficult, get the front leg into position and allow the back leg to be wherever it works for you. Once your body gets used to that shape, try moving the back leg into a 90-degree angle.

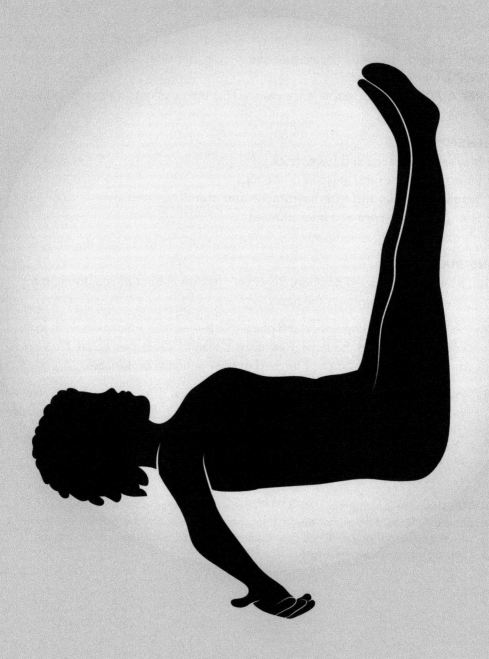

LEGS UP THE WALL POSE
VIPARITA KARANI

TIME: Remain in the pose for 5 to 20 minutes.

PROPS: Strap, sandbag, or heavy blanket

PRECAUTIONS: Those with eye injuries or head injuries and those in the second and third trimesters of pregnancy should avoid this pose. For sacroiliac joint or hamstring injuries, modify by resting the calves on the seat of a chair or a couch with bent knees.

BENEFITS:
- Relieves lower-back pain
- Loosens the leg muscles for more flexibility in movement
- Relaxes the nervous system
- May improve circulation and lymphatic drainage

INSTRUCTIONS:
1. Sit with your right hip against a wall. Place your hands behind you. Simultaneously slide your legs up the wall while rotating both hips toward the wall and lie on your back. Or lie on your side with your hips against the wall and knees squeezed into the chest; then roll onto your back, sliding your legs up the wall.

2. Scoot your hips as close to the wall as possible. Relax your arms out by your sides, release all tension, and close your eyes.

3. To exit the pose, bend your knees, roll onto your side, and then press up to seated.

TIP: If adding a blanket or sandbag, once your legs are up the wall, bend your knees and place the prop on your feet, or have someone place it for you. If using a strap, secure it around your ankles before entering the pose.

CHAPTER 5

THE SEQUENCES

The sequences in this chapter will help you build a home yoga practice and reach your flexibility goals. Each sequence includes a list of poses and instructions for transitioning between the poses and states how long to hold each pose.

Familiarize yourself with each pose before attempting the sequence, especially if you have any injuries. See each individual pose page for specific instructions, modifications, and tips related to the pose.

WAKE-UP FLOW

TIME: 25 to 45 minutes

REPETITIONS: None

PROPS: Blanket, blocks

PRECAUTIONS: If you have a knee injury, try modifying for Child's Pose. If you have a back injury, keep your back straight in Half Split and Seated Forward Bend.

BENEFITS:
- Great for stretching your whole body for a morning energy boost
- Stretches the hips, hamstrings, shoulders, and back
- Strengthens the legs, shoulders, back, and core

INSTRUCTIONS

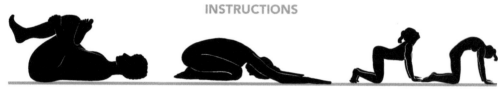

1. Start in **Reclined Figure-Four Pose** (page 93). Hold for 5 to 10 deep breaths on each side.

2. Roll to one side and sit back into **Child's Pose** (page 87). Hold for two to five minutes. Walk your hands side to side.

3. Come to tabletop and move through three to eight rounds of **Cat-Cow** (page 33).

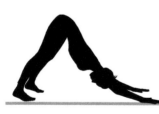
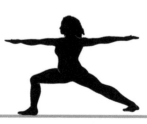
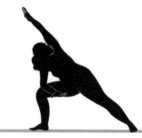

4. Lift your hips into **Downward-Facing Dog** (page 31). Hold for five deep breaths.

5. Step your right foot forward for **Warrior II** (page 61). Hold for five deep breaths.

6. Lower your right forearm for **Extended Side Angle** (page 63). Hold for five deep breaths.

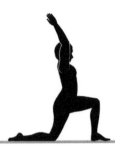
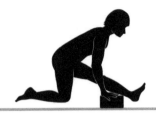
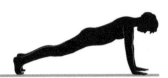

7. Place your hands on either side of your right foot, lower your left knee, and lift into **Low Lunge** (page 35). Hold for five deep breaths.

8. Straighten your right leg for **Half Split** (page 55). Hold for five deep breaths.

9. Step your right foot back and into **Plank Pose** (page 27). Hold for one or more deep breaths.

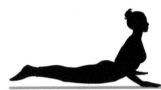
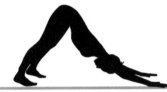

10. Lower to your belly for **Cobra Pose** (page 29). Take one deep breath, and then lower your chest.

11. Press back up into **Downward-Facing Dog** (page 31).

12. Repeat **Warrior II**, **Extended Side Angle** (page 63), **Low Lunge** (page 35), and **Half Split** (page 55) on the other side.

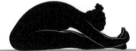

13. Repeat **Plank Pose** (page 27), **Cobra Pose** (page 29), and **Downward-Facing Dog** (page 31).

14. Come into **Seated Forward Bend** (page 45). Hold for 5 to 10 deep breaths.

TIP: This sequence can be lengthened by repeating Warrior II, Extended Side Angle, Low Lunge, and Half Split a few times on each side. Add Plank, Cobra Pose, and Downward-Facing Dog in between sides to create a flow.

MORNING MOBILITY SUN SALUTATION

TIME: 10 to 20 minutes
REPETITIONS: Repeat five times or as many as desired.
PROPS: None
PRECAUTIONS: Do not practice Standing Forward Fold or Downward-Facing Dog if you have eye or head injuries. Practice on an empty stomach or you may experience heartburn or indigestion. If you have wrist injuries, shoulder injuries, or spinal injuries, use caution and modify for Standing Forward Fold, Plank Pose, Cobra Pose, and Downward-Facing Dog. If you have high blood pressure, consult your doctor before attempting this sequence.

BENEFITS:
- Boosts energy and increases blood flow
- Can be used as a warm-up before other sequences or as a stand-alone practice
- Strengthens the core, shoulders, and back
- Improves flexibility of the hamstrings, chest, and spine
- Helps improve posture

INSTRUCTIONS

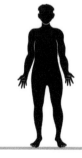 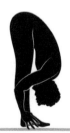 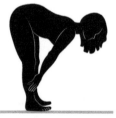

1. Stand at the top of your mat in **Mountain Pose** (page 21).

2. Inhale and reach your arms up. Exhale, hinge from your hips, and fold into **Standing Forward Fold** (page 23).

3. Inhale, place your hands on your shins, and lengthen your spine for **Standing Half Forward Fold** (page 25).

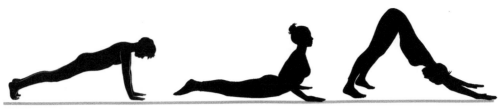

4. Exhale, lower your hands down, and step back to **Plank Pose** (page 27). Lower down to the mat. Set your knees down first for support if needed.

5. Inhale and come into **Cobra Pose** (page 29).

6. Exhale, press into your hands, and push up, either back to **Plank Pose** (page 27) or onto your hands and knees. Lift your hips into **Downward-Facing Dog** (page 31). Hold for five deep breaths.

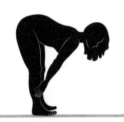

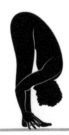

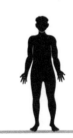

7. Walk or lightly hop your feet to the top of the mat just behind your hands. Inhale and return to **Standing Half Forward Fold** (page 25).

8. Exhale, fold forward, and place your hands on the mat for **Standing Forward Fold** (page 23).

9. Inhale, bend your knees slightly, and rise to stand, reaching arms up overhead. Exhale and lower hands by the sides to come back to **Mountain Pose** (page 21).

TIP: This sequence is great first thing in the morning. Put your yoga mat by your bed so you can do a few rounds when you first wake up to get energized for the day! If using this sequence as a stand-alone practice, end with a few minutes in Corpse Pose (page 51).

WIND-DOWN SEQUENCE

TIME: 40 to 60 minutes

REPETITIONS: None

PROPS: Block, bolster, or stack of blankets

PRECAUTIONS: Those with eye or head injuries should avoid Legs Up the Wall Pose and practice Corpse Pose (page 51) instead. If you have a back injury, fold with a straight spine in Head-to-Knee Pose.

BENEFITS:

- Relaxes the nervous system to help you sleep
- Stretches the neck, legs, spine, back, and hips
- May help reduce neck and back pain

INSTRUCTIONS

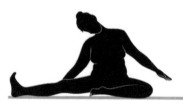
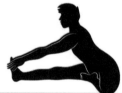
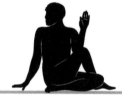

1. Begin seated and come into **Seated Neck Release Pose** (page 83). Hold for five deep breaths, or longer if desired.

2. Place your hands on either side of your right leg and fold forward for **Head-to-Knee Pose** (page 43). Hold for 5 to 10 deep breaths.

3. Lift your torso and cross your left foot over your right thigh for **Half Lord of the Fishes** (page 85). Hold for 5 to 10 deep breaths.

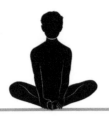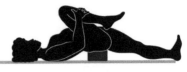

4. Place the soles of your feet together and open your knees into **Bound Angle Pose** (page 39). Hold for 5 to 10 deep breaths.

5. Place your right foot against your left inner thigh and repeat **Seated Neck Release Pose** (page 83), **Head-to-Knee Pose** (page 43), and **Half Lord of the Fishes** (page 85) on the other side.

6. Grab a prop and lie on your back for **Psoas Release Pose** (page 97). Hold for two to five minutes on each side.

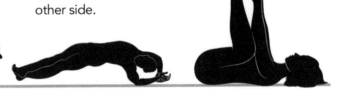

7. Remove the prop and lower your hips to the mat. Pull your knees into your chest and lower them to the right for **Supine Twist** (page 89). Hold for two to five minutes on each side.

8. Extend your legs and set up for **Banana Pose** (page 95). Hold for two to five minutes on each side.

9. Pull your knees into your chest and move into **Happy Baby** (page 47). Hold for 5 to 10 deep breaths, or longer if desired.

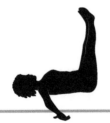

10. End your practice with 5 to 20 minutes in **Legs Up the Wall Pose** (page 103).

TIP: This sequence is perfect right before bed to help you unwind from your day, but it can be practiced anytime you want to stretch and release tension. Hold the poses longer and add as many props as you'd like to make this practice more restful.

MEDITATIVE MOON SALUTATION

TIME: 10 to 20 minutes
REPETITIONS: Repeat this sequence five times or as many as desired.
PROPS: Blocks or thick books
PRECAUTIONS: Use caution in Yogi Squat if you have a knee injury.

BENEFITS:
- Great for those who are pregnant or unable to bear weight in their arms
- Stretches the hips, legs, and spine
- Strengthens the legs, hips, and core
- Improves balance and posture

INSTRUCTIONS

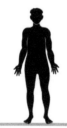 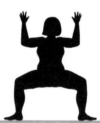 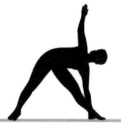

1. Stand at the top of your mat in **Mountain Pose** (page 21).

2. Inhale and step your right foot to the right so feet are wide and come into **Goddess Pose** (page 59).

3. Exhale, straighten your legs, and pivot your left toes to face the top of the mat and your right toes to face the top right corner of the mat for **Triangle Pose** (page 65).

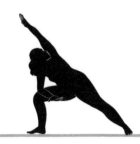
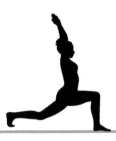
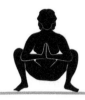

4. Inhale and bend your left knee, placing your left forearm onto your left thigh for **Extended Side Angle** (page 63). Exhale and lower your right arm.

5. Inhale, lift your torso, rotate your chest to face forward, and move into **Crescent Lunge** (page 57).

6. Exhale and lower your hands to the inside of your left foot. Step your right foot outside your right hand for **Yogi Squat** (page 67).

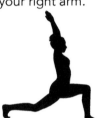
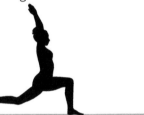
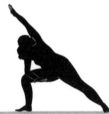

7. Inhale, step your left foot back, and lift your torso into **Crescent Lunge** (page 57) on the other side.

8. Exhale, bend your right knee, and place your right forearm on your right thigh for **Extended Side Angle** (page 63) on the other side.

9. Inhale and straighten your right leg to transition into **Triangle Pose** (page 65) on the other side.

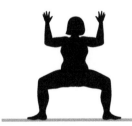
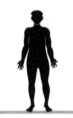

10. Exhale and transition to **Goddess Pose** (page 59).

11. Inhale, and step your left foot forward to **Mountain Pose** (page 21).

TIP: Make this sequence more cardiovascular by staying for only one breath in each pose, or build strength by holding the poses for longer periods. Be sure to switch which leg you step back with from Mountain Pose each time you repeat.

LOWER-BACK RESCUE

TIME: 25 to 40 minutes
REPETITIONS: None
PROPS: Block or stack of folded blankets; blanket
PRECAUTIONS: If you have sciatica or knee injuries, practice Star-Shaped Pigeon (page 101) instead of Pigeon Pose. If you have spinal injuries, practice cautiously and use modifications for Camel Pose.

BENEFITS:
- Improves hip, hamstring, and spinal flexibility to help relieve lower-back pain
- Strengthens the hips, back, core, and legs
- Improves posture and moves the spine in all directions

INSTRUCTIONS

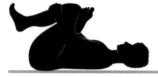 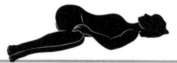 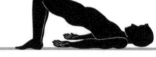

1. Lie on your back with knees bent and come into **Reclined Figure-Four Pose** (page 93). Hold for five deep breaths on each side.

2. Uncross your ankle and transition into **Supine Twist** (page 89). Stay for 5 to 10 deep breaths on each side.

3. Lower your feet to the floor for **Bridge Pose** (page 91). Hold for three to five breaths.

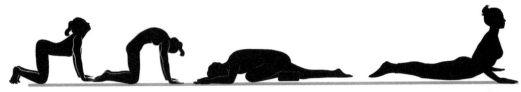

4. Lower your hips, roll to one side, and push up to tabletop. Move through three to five rounds of **Cat-Cow** (page 33).

5. Slide your right knee forward and come into **Pigeon Pose** (page 69). Hold for 5 to 10 breaths.

6. Come back to table-top, lower onto your belly, and inhale as you lift into **Cobra Pose** (page 29).

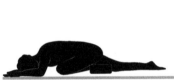

7. Exhale and lower back down. Press onto your hands and knees and repeat **Pigeon Pose** (page 69) on the opposite side.

8. Return to hands and knees, and then come into **Camel Pose** (page 71) for five breaths.

9. Sit and extend your right leg to come into **Head-to-Knee Pose** (page 43). Hold for 5 to 10 deep breaths, and then repeat on the other side.

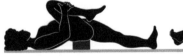

10. Grab a prop and lie on back for **Psoas Release Pose** (page 97). Hold for 2 to 10 minutes on each side.

11. Remove the prop and lower your hips. Transition into **Banana Pose** (page 95). Hold for one to five minutes on each side.

TIP: In backbends like Camel Pose and Cobra Pose, focus on length-ening the spine rather than pushing to a deeper backbend. Repeat these poses a few times, gradually increasing the backbend each time.

HIPS AND SHOULDERS RESCUE

TIME: 30 to 45 minutes

REPETITIONS: None

PROPS: Block or stack of blankets

PRECAUTIONS: For neck injuries, move slowly into Seated Neck Release and Fish Pose, and if you experience any tingling or numbness, back out of the stretch. If you have a knee injury, modify Yogi Squat by sitting on a block or blankets.

BENEFITS:

- Counters the effects of sitting
- Relaxes the nervous system
- Relieves tension in the shoulders, neck, hips, and back
- Stretches the neck, shoulders, back, chest, spine, legs, and hips
- May help relieve headaches, insomnia, pain from menstrual cramps

---

INSTRUCTIONS

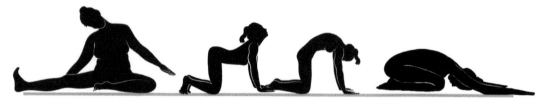

1. Sit with your right leg extended for **Seated Neck Release Pose** (page 83). Hold for 5 to 10 breaths, and then repeat on the other side.

2. Come to tabletop. Move through 5 to 10 rounds of **Cat-Cow** (page 33).

3. Bring your big toes together, widen your knees, and sink into **Child's Pose** (page 87). Hold for three to eight minutes.

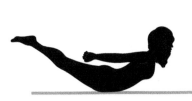 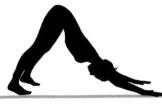

4. Come back to tabletop, and then lower onto your belly for **Bound Locust** (page 81). Hold for three to five breaths.

5. Push up onto your hands and knees and come into **Downward-Facing Dog** (page 31). Hold for three to five breaths.

6. Walk your feet outside your hands to transition into **Yogi Squat** (page 67). Stay for one to two minutes. Place your hands out in front and walk feet back to come to hands and knees.

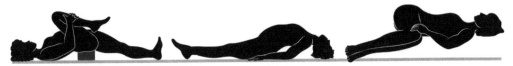

7. Grab a prop and lie back. Spend two to five minutes per side in **Psoas Release Pose** (page 97).

8. Remove the prop and lower your hips to transition into **Fish Pose** (page 49). Stay for 5 to 10 breaths.

9. Lie down, pull your knees into your chest, and come into **Supine Twist** (page 89). Stay for one to five minutes per side.

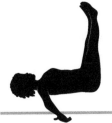

10. End your practice with 5 to 10 minutes in **Legs Up the Wall Pose** (page 103).

TIP: In Child's Pose, try walking your hands as far to one side as you can, letting your rib cage drop toward the floor to stretch the sides of the upper back. Repeat on the other side.

TECH-NECK RESCUE

TIME: 25 to 40 minutes
REPETITIONS: None
PROPS: Blanket, strap
PRECAUTIONS: If you have a back injury, keep your backbends mild and focus on lengthening your spine in Puppy Pose, Bound Locust Pose, and Camel Pose.

BENEFITS:
• Stretches the neck, spine, chest, shoulders, and hips
• Strengthens the upper back
• May reduce neck pain and headaches
• Improves posture and counters the effects of sitting

INSTRUCTIONS

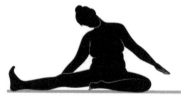 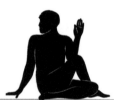

1. Sit with your right leg extended for **Seated Neck Release Pose** (page 83). Hold for five deep breaths.

2. Cross your left foot over the right thigh to transition into **Half Lord of the Fishes** (page 85). Hold for 5 to 10 deep breaths.

3. Stack your knees and transition to **Cow Face Pose** (page 41). Hold for five deep breaths.

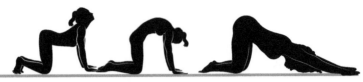

4. Repeat **Seated Neck Release Pose** (page 83), **Half Lord of the Fishes** (page 85), and **Cow Face Pose** (page 41) on the other side.

5. Uncross your legs, place your hands in front of you, and come to tabletop. Move through three to five rounds of **Cat-Cow** (page 33).

6. Walk your hands forward and lower your chest into **Puppy Pose** (page 75). Hold for 5 to 10 deep breaths.

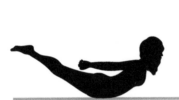

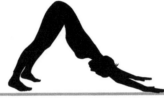

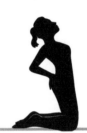

7. Lower onto your belly for **Bound Locust Pose** (page 81). Hold for three to eight deep breaths.

8. Place your hands under your shoulders, push up to tabletop, and lift the hips into **Downward-Facing Dog** (page 31).

9. Lower your knees onto the mat or a blanket for **Camel Pose** (page 71). Hold for five deep breaths and repeat two or three times if desired.

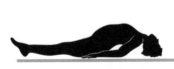

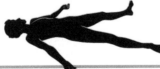

10. Lie on your back to transition into **Fish Pose** (page 49). Hold for five to eight deep breaths.

11. End your practice with 5 to 10 minutes in **Corpse Pose** (page 51).

TIP: If you use a computer or a phone for long periods of time, try doing modifications of these poses in a chair throughout the day: Seated Neck Release, Half Lord of the Fishes, Cow Face Pose, Cat-Cow, and Bound Locust Pose.

SITTING RESCUE

TIME: 20 to 30 minutes

REPETITIONS: This sequence can be done once or repeated from Cat-Cow to Camel Pose a few times for a longer practice.

PROPS: Block or stack of blankets

PRECAUTIONS: If you have an eye or head injury, avoid Downward-Facing Dog. If your knees are sensitive, pad them with a blanket in Cat-Cow, Low Lunge, and Camel Pose.

BENEFITS:

• Improves posture and counters the effects of sitting
• Stretches the hip flexors, spine, core, legs, and chest
• Strengthens the back, core, and legs

INSTRUCTIONS

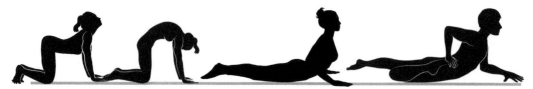

1. Begin in tabletop. Move through three to eight rounds of **Cat-Cow** (page 33).

2. Lower onto your belly for **Cobra Pose** (page 29). Hold for one to three deep breaths.

3. Place your elbows under your shoulders to transition into **Half Frog Pose** (page 99). Hold for five deep breaths on each side.

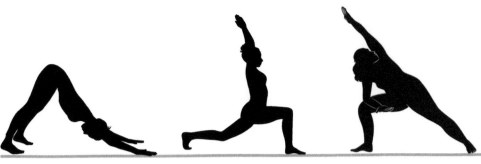

4. Lower your chest and transition into **Downward-Facing Dog** (page 31). Hold for three to five breaths.

5. Step your right foot between your hands to transition into **Crescent Lunge** (page 57). Hold for five deep breaths.

6. Lower the left heel, place the right forearm on the right thigh, and come into **Extended Side Angle** (page 63). Hold for five deep breaths.

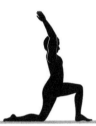

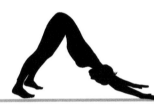

7. Place your hands on either side of your right foot, lower your left knee, and lift into **Low Lunge** (page 35). Hold for five deep breaths.

8. Lower your hands to the mat and step your right foot back into **Downward-Facing Dog** (page 31).

9. Repeat **Crescent Lunge** (page 57), **Extended Side Angle** (page 63), and **Low Lunge** (page 35) on the other side.

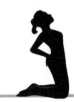

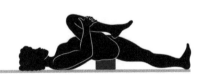

10. Place your hands on the mat and step your left foot back for **Camel Pose** (page 71). Hold for three to five deep breaths.

11. Grab a prop, and lie back to transition into **Psoas Release Pose** (page 97). Hold for two to five minutes on each side.

TIP: To accentuate the hip flexor stretch in Half Frog Pose, press your hip bones into the mat.

SAY GOODBYE TO SCIATICA

TIME: 30 to 60 minutes
REPETITIONS: None
PROPS: Block or thick books
PRECAUTIONS: Work within a pain-free range of motion and do not force your body into a deeper stretch, as it may reinjure the sciatic nerve.

BENEFITS:
• Helps relieve sciatica pain by stretching the hamstrings, hips, and spine
• Prevents sciatica flare-ups by strengthening the core, back muscles, and hips

INSTRUCTIONS

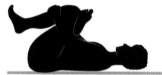 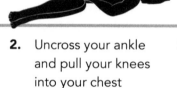

1. Lie on your back with knees bent for **Reclined Figure-Four Pose** (page 93). Hold for one to five minutes on each side.

2. Uncross your ankle and pull your knees into your chest for **Supine Twist** (page 89). Hold for one to five minutes on each side.

3. Ground your feet and lift hips into **Bridge Pose** (page 91). Hold for one to four minutes.

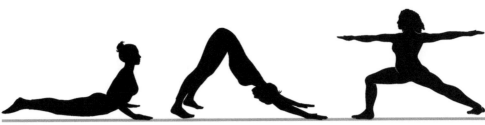

4. Roll onto your belly. Inhale, pull your chest up into **Cobra Pose** (page 29), and exhale to lower. Repeat 3 to 10 times.

5. Press up into table-top, and then lift your hips into **Downward-Facing Dog** (page 31). Bend the knees slightly and hold for three to five breaths.

6. Step your right foot forward and stand up for **Warrior II** (page 61). Hold for three to eight breaths, and then switch sides by adjusting the feet.

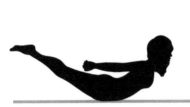
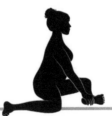
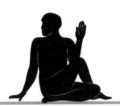

7. Lower onto your belly for **Bound Locust** (page 81). Hold for two to five deep breaths.

8. Press up to table-top, sit on the mat, and move into **Star-Shaped Pigeon** (page 101). Hold the pose for 5 to 10 breaths on each side.

9. Return to seated to transition into **Half Lord of the Fishes** (page 85). Hold for 5 to 10 breaths per side.

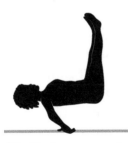

10. End your practice with 2 to 10 minutes in **Legs Up the Wall Pose** (page 103).

TIP: Mild backbends like Bridge Pose, Cobra Pose, and Bound Locust can be beneficial for sciatica when you focus on lengthening the spine rather than pushing yourself into a deep backbend.

TIME: 25 to 35 minutes

REPETITIONS: None

PROPS: Block or stack of blankets

PRECAUTIONS: If you have a knee injury, practice Yogi Squat with a pain-free range of motion, adding a block under the hips for support if desired. Do not practice Downward-Facing Dog or Bridge Pose if you have an eye or head injury.

BENEFITS:

- Stretches the hips, hamstrings, core, and spine
- Relieves tension from the lower back and may reduce back pain and menstrual cramps
- May help improve digestion

INSTRUCTIONS

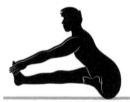 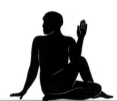

1. Sit with your right leg straight out for **Head-to-Knee Pose** (page 43). Hold for 5 to 10 deep breaths.

2. Lift your torso and cross your left foot over right thigh to transition into **Half Lord of the Fishes** (page 85). Hold for 5 to 10 deep breaths.

3. Repeat **Head-to-Knee Pose** (page 43) and **Half Lord of the Fishes** (page 85) on the other side.

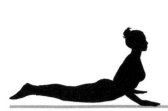 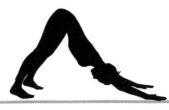 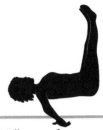

4. Come to tabletop, and then lower onto your belly for **Cobra Pose** (page 29). Repeat three to five times.

5. Place your hands under your shoulders, press to tabletop, and lift your hips into **Downward-Facing Dog** (page 31). Hold for three to five breaths.

6. Walk your feet outside your hands and lower the hips into **Yogi Squat** (page 67). Stay for one to three minutes. Place hands out in front and walk feet back to come to tabletop.

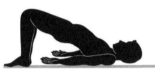 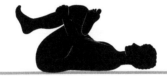 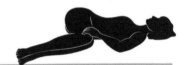

7. Lie on your back for **Bridge Pose** (page 91). Hold for 5 to 10 deep breaths.

8. Lower your hips and transition into **Reclined Figure-Four Pose** (page 93). Hold for 5 to 10 deep breaths on each side.

9. Uncross your legs and pull your knees into your chest for **Supine Twist** (page 89). Hold for 5 to 10 deep breaths, and then repeat on the other side.

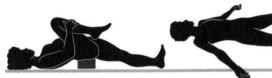

10. Grab a prop and place it under the hips for **Psoas Release Pose** (page 97). Hold for two to five minutes on each side.

11. Remove the prop and lower your hips. End your practice with 5 to 10 minutes in **Corpse Pose** (page 51).

TIP: This sequence is also great for digestion and can be done after a big meal like a holiday dinner.

LOVE YOUR SPINE

TIME: 25 to 40 minutes
REPETITIONS: None
PROPS: Blanket, strap
PRECAUTIONS: Skip Downward-Facing Dog if you have an eye or head injury.

BENEFITS:
- Stretches the spine, side body, shoulders, arms, legs, and hips
- Improves posture and counters the effects of sitting
- Moves the spine in all directions to improve range of motion
- May help reduce back pain
- Improves twisting range of motion, which can improve athletic performance in sports, such as golf and baseball

---

INSTRUCTIONS

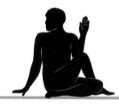

1. Begin seated and cross your right leg over the left thigh to set up for **Half Lord of the Fishes** (page 85). Hold for five deep breaths.

2. Stack your knees for **Cow Face Pose** (page 41). Hold for five deep breaths.

3. Repeat **Half Lord of the Fishes** (page 85) and **Cow Face Pose** (page 41) on the other side.

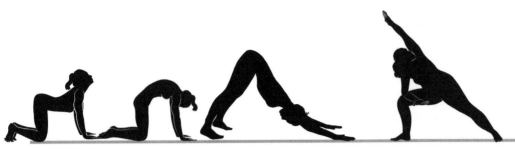

4. Come to table-top and move through three to five rounds of **Cat-Cow** (page 33).

5. Tuck your toes and lift your hips into **Downward-Facing Dog** (page 31). Hold for three to five deep breaths.

6. Step your right foot between your hands and stand up for **Extended Side Angle** (page 63). Hold for five deep breaths.

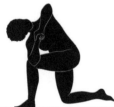

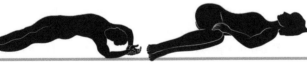

7. Lower your left knee, lift your torso, and come into **Lunge Twist** (page 37). Hold for five deep breaths.

8. Unwind, lower your hands to the mat, and step your right foot back for **Downward-Facing Dog** (page 31).

9. Repeat **Extended Side Angle** (page 63) and **Lunge Twist** (page 37) on the other side.

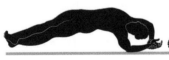

10. Return to tabletop, and then lie on your back for **Banana Pose** (page 95). Hold for two to five minutes per side.

11. Draw your knees in and drop them to the right for **Supine Twist** (page 89). Hold for 5 to 10 breaths; repeat on the other side.

12. End your practice with 5 to 10 minutes in **Corpse Pose** (page 51).

TIP: Breathe as you twist. Inhale to lengthen the spine, and exhale as you deepen the twist, especially in Half Lord of the Fishes and Lunge Twist.

OPEN YOUR HEART

TIME: 30 to 40 minutes
REPETITIONS: None
PROPS: Blanket, block or thick books
PRECAUTIONS: If you have a spinal injury, move slowly into your backbends and twists, and focus on maintaining a long spine.

BENEFITS:
• Stretches the chest, triceps, spine, hips, and legs
• Strengthens the upper back, shoulders, core, hips, and legs
• Helps improve posture and counters the effects of sitting
• May help reduce shoulder, back, and neck pain, and headaches

---

INSTRUCTIONS

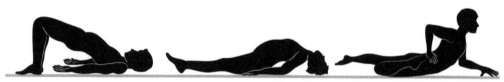

1. Lie on your back with your knees bent for **Bridge Pose** (page 91). Hold for five deep breaths.

2. Lower your hips, extend your legs, and come into **Fish Pose** (page 49). Stay for five to eight breaths.

3. Flip over onto your belly for **Half Frog Pose** (page 99). Take five breaths on each side.

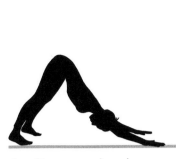
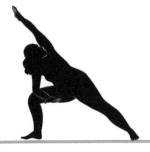
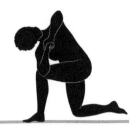

4. Place your hands under your shoulders, press up to tabletop, and then lift your hips into **Downward-Facing Dog** (page 31). Hold for three to five deep breaths.

5. Step your right foot between your hands and move into **Extended Side Angle** (page 63) for five deep breaths.

6. Lower your hands on either side of your right foot, set your left knee down, and come into **Lunge Twist** (page 37) for five deep breaths.

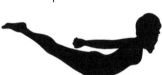
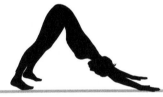
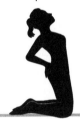

7. Place your hands down, step your right foot back, and lower onto your belly for **Bound Locust** (page 81). Hold for three to five breaths.

8. Push up to tabletop, and return to **Downward-Facing Dog** (page 31). Then repeat **Extended Side Angle** (page 63) and **Lunge Twist** (page 37) on the left side.

9. Place your hands down and slide your left knee back to meet the right. Kneel for **Camel Pose** (page 71). Hold for five deep breaths.

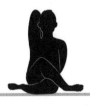
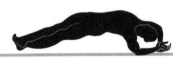

10. Come to a seated position to transition into **Cow Face Pose** (page 41). Hold for five to eight breaths on each side.

11. Lie on your back and come into **Banana Pose** (page 95). Hold for two to five minutes on each side.

TIP: In Fish Pose, Extended Side Angle, and Bound Locust, squeeze your shoulder blades together and breathe deeply into the chest to help relax and stretch it.

UNLOCK YOUR SHOULDERS

TIME: 40 to 50 minutes

REPETITIONS: None

PRECAUTIONS: If you have shoulder injuries, check with your doctor before attempting this sequence.

BENEFITS:
- Strengthens the shoulders, core, and back muscles
- Stretches the shoulders, neck, and chest
- Improves shoulder mobility for pain relief and injury prevention
- Improves athletic performance for activities like weight training and sports like tennis, baseball, volleyball, and basketball

INSTRUCTIONS

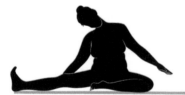 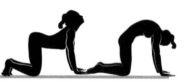

1. Sit with your right leg extended for **Seated Neck Release Pose** (page 83). Hold for five deep breaths, and then repeat on the other side.

2. Cross your right leg over your left leg and set up for **Cow Face Pose** (page 41). Hold for 5 to 10 breaths on each side.

3. Come to tabletop and move through 5 to 10 rounds of **Cat-Cow** (page 33).

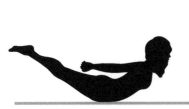

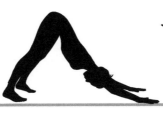

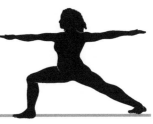

4. Lower onto your belly for **Bound Locust** (page 81). Hold for five breaths.

5. Press up to tabletop and lift your hips into **Downward-Facing Dog** (page 31). Hold for five deep breaths.

6. Step your right foot between your hands and stand for **Warrior II** (page 61). Hold for five deep breaths.

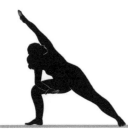

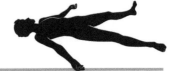

7. Lower your right forearm onto your right thigh for **Extended Side Angle** (page 63). Hold for five deep breaths.

8. Lift your torso and switch the position of the legs. Then repeat **Warrior II** (page 61) and **Extended Side Angle** (page 63) on the other side.

9. Lower your hands onto the mat, set the knees down, and come into **Puppy Pose** (page 75). Hold for 5 to 10 breaths.

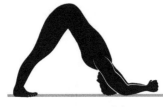

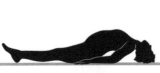

10. Press up to tabletop, lower your forearms onto the mat, and come into **Dolphin Pose** (page 77). Hold for 5 to 10 deep breaths.

11. Lower your knees, and then lie on your back for **Fish Pose** (page 49). Hold for 5 to 10 deep breaths.

12. End your practice with five minutes or more in **Corpse Pose** (page 51).

TIP: Breathe deeply into your chest and shoulders as you move through the poses in this sequence to get the most out of each stretch.

INVERT YOUR WORLD

TIME: 25 to 30 minutes

REPETITIONS: None

PROPS: None

PRECAUTIONS: Avoid inversions if you have an eye or head injury. If you have a wrist injury, use caution or modifications when bearing weight on your hands.

BENEFITS:
- Strengthens the shoulders, legs, and core
- Stretches the back, shoulders, chest, legs, and core
- May help boost energy and reduce fatigue

INSTRUCTIONS

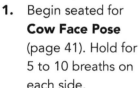 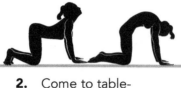

1. Begin seated for **Cow Face Pose** (page 41). Hold for 5 to 10 breaths on each side.

2. Come to table-top and move through three to five rounds of **Cat-Cow** (page 33).

3. Walk your hands forward for **Puppy Pose** (page 75). Hold for 5 to 10 breaths.

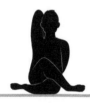 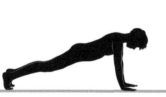 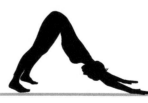 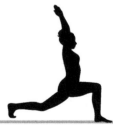

4. Walk your hands under the shoulders and come into **Plank Pose** (page 27). Hold for three to five deep breaths.

5. Lift your hips into **Downward-Facing Dog** (page 31). Hold for five deep breaths.

6. Step your right foot forward and lift up for **Crescent Lunge** (page 57). Hold for five deep breaths.

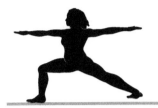 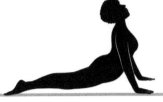 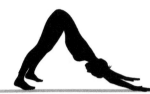

7. Ground your left heel down and open your arms out into **Warrior II** (page 61). Hold for five deep breaths.

8. Place your hands down, step back into **Plank Pose** (page 27), then come into **Upward-Facing Dog** (page 73). Hold for one to three breaths.

9. Lift your hips and tuck your toes to return to **Downward-Facing Dog** (page 31).

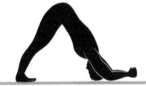

10. Repeat **Crescent Lunge** (page 57) and **Warrior II** (page 61) on the other side.

11. Repeat **Plank Pose**, **Upward-Facing Dog** (page 73), and **Downward-Facing Dog** (page 31), and then set your knees down.

12. Place your forearms down for **Dolphin Pose** (page 77). Hold for 5 to 10 breaths.

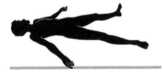

13. Lower to your knees, and then lie on your back to end your practice with five minutes in **Corpse Pose** (page 51).

TIP: Dolphin Pose serves as this sequence's peak pose, meaning that the poses before it prepare your body for this more intense inversion. In gentler poses like Puppy Pose and Plank Pose, focus on engaging your muscles so that when you get to Dolphin Pose you're warmed up and ready.

LOWER-BODY LOVE

TIME: 30 to 45 minutes
REPETITIONS: None
PROPS: Block or stack of blankets
PRECAUTIONS: If you have a spinal injury, keep your back straight in forward folds, such as Head-to-Knee Pose and Half Split. If you have sciatica or knee injuries, practice Star-Shaped Pigeon (page 101) instead of Pigeon Pose.

BENEFITS:
- Stretches the hips, hamstrings, calves, and lower back
- Strengthens the legs and hips
- Helps relieve pain and tension in the lower back and hips and counters the effects of sitting

---

INSTRUCTIONS

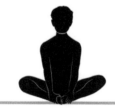 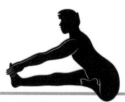 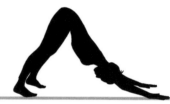

1. Begin seated with feet together in **Bound Angle Pose** (page 39). Stay for 5 to 10 breaths.

2. Extend your right leg for **Head-to-Knee Pose** (page 43). Stay for five breaths. Repeat on the other side.

3. Come to tabletop. Lift your hips into **Downward-Facing Dog** (page 31). Stay for one to two breaths.

■ **TIP:** Try adding movement in Happy Baby by swaying from side to side if you'd like.

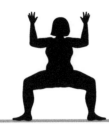 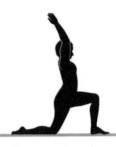 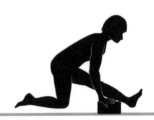

4. Step your right foot forward to transition to **Goddess Pose** (page 59). Take five deep breaths.

5. Set your hands on either side of your right foot and lower your left knee for **Low Lunge** (page 35). Hold for five breaths.

6. Transition into **Half Split** (page 55) by straightening your right leg. Hold for five breaths.

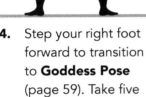 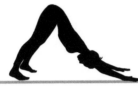

7. Transition into **Pigeon Pose** (page 69) by lowering your shin down. Hold for one to three minutes.

8. Transition back into **Downward-Facing Dog** (page 31) by stepping your right leg back.

9. Repeat **Goddess Pose** (page 59), **Low Lunge** (page 35), **Half Split** (page 55), and **Pigeon Pose** (page 69) with the left foot forward.

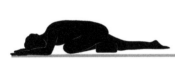 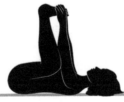 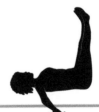

10. Sit onto your left hip, grab a prop, and lie back for **Psoas Release Pose** (page 97). Hold for two to five minutes on each side.

11. Remove the prop for **Happy Baby** (page 47). Hold for 5 to 10 deep breaths.

12. End your practice with 5 to 10 minutes in **Legs Up the Wall Pose** (page 103).

FOLD INTO PEACE

TIME: 30 to 40 minutes

REPETITIONS: None

PROPS: Block or stack of blankets

PRECAUTIONS: If you have sciatica or a knee injury, practice Star-Shaped Pigeon (page 101) instead of Pigeon Pose. Those with knee injuries should also use caution with Child's Pose.

BENEFITS:
- Stretches the legs, back, and hips
- Relaxes the nervous system to help relieve stress and insomnia

---

INSTRUCTIONS

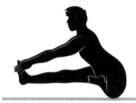 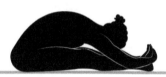 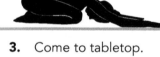

1. Begin seated with your right leg straight for **Head-to-Knee Pose** (page 43). Hold for 5 to 10 deep breaths on each side.

2. Straighten your legs and come into **Seated Forward Bend** (page 45). Hold for 5 to 10 deep breaths.

3. Come to tabletop. Transition to **Child's Pose** (page 87) and hold for two to five minutes.

TIP: Forward folds are naturally introspective. Close eyes and breathe deeply to relax into these poses, rather than pushing yourself into a deeper stretch.

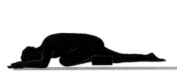
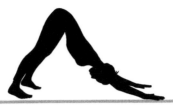
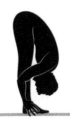

4. Press up and slide your right shin forward into **Pigeon Pose** (page 69). Hold for two to five minutes, and then repeat on the other side.

5. Lift back to tabletop, and then come into **Downward-Facing Dog** (page 31). Hold for three to eight deep breaths.

6. Walk your feet to the hands to come into **Standing Forward Fold** (page 23). Hold for five deep breaths.

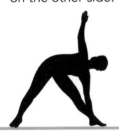
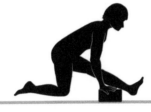
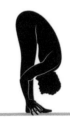

7. Step your left foot back and stand for **Triangle Pose** (page 65). Hold for five deep breaths.

8. Place your hands on the mat, lower your left knee, and straighten your right leg for **Half Split** (page 55). Hold for five deep breaths.

9. Bend your right knee and step your left foot forward to return to **Standing Forward Fold** (page 23).

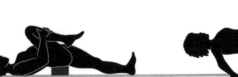

10. Step your right foot back and repeat **Triangle Pose** (page 65) and **Half Split** (page 55) on other side.

11. Come to tabletop. Then grab a prop and lie on your back for **Psoas Release Pose** (page 97). Hold for two to five minutes on each side.

12. Remove the prop and end your practice with 5 to 10 minutes in **Legs Up the Wall Pose** (page 103).

Build Your Own Sequence

Building your own sequence can be a fun and creative way to give your body exactly what it needs based on your flexibility goals. Use the preceding sequences as a starting point and add others, or start from scratch to build something new.

If you're building a sequence from scratch, start with warm-up poses to prepare your body for deeper stretches. These can be seated, like Seated Neck Release or Bound Angle Pose, or start with Child's Pose or Cat-Cow.

You don't need to create a flow, as in traditional Sun or Moon Salutations, but it's good to consider your transitions from one pose to the next. If you want to do Downward-Facing Dog, Triangle Pose, Cobra Pose, Warrior II, Low Lunge, Camel Pose, and Bridge Pose, try ordering them so you don't have to go from standing to lying down and then back to standing again. Try this:

- Warrior II

- Triangle Pose

- Low Lunge

- Cobra Pose

- Downward-Facing Dog

- Warrior II, Triangle, and Low Lunge on the other side

- Camel Pose

- Bridge Pose

Some yoga sequences build to a peak pose. In the Invert Your World sequence, for example, Dolphin Pose is the peak pose. This means Dolphin is the most intense and complex pose of the sequence. The poses that come before the peak properly warm and prepare your body for it. If you want to build to Yogi Squat, place poses that stretch the hips, calves, and hamstrings before it (like Half Split, Triangle Pose, and Warrior II).

Your sequences should build an energy arc. They should start with less intense and simpler poses to warm your body, build intensity with deeper stretches or more challenging poses, and then wind down into cooldown poses.

Also think about adding counterposes. If you're practicing a lot of backbends, like Camel Pose and Puppy Pose, counter them with poses to help neutralize your spine afterward. This could be a pose with a straight spine, like Downward-Facing Dog, or a twisting pose, like Half Lord of the Fishes or Supine Twist. To counter hip-opening poses, like Goddess Pose and Bound Angle Pose, which involve external rotation, add a pose with internal rotation, like Cow Face Pose or Half Lord of the Fishes.

Add the Morning Mobility Sun Salutation and Meditative Moon Salutation sequences to your own sequences for a full hour-long practice. Begin with some warm-ups, do a few rounds of Sun or Moon Salutations, and then finish with cooldown poses.

Always end your practice with a few minutes in a restful pose, like Corpse Pose or Legs Up the Wall Pose.

RESOURCES

Books

Fierce Medicine: Breakthrough Practices to Heal the Body and Ignite the Spirit by Ana Forrest

Chronicles the life of Ana Forrest and her healing journey through yoga, providing poses and exercises to try in your own yoga practice.

The Path of the Yoga Sutras: A Practical Guide to the Core of Yoga by Nicolai Bachman

An easy-to-understand approach for those who are interested in learning about yoga philosophy.

The Power of Ashtanga Yoga: Developing a Practice That Will Bring You Strength, Flexibility, and Inner Peace by Kino MacGregor

A guide for learning Ashtanga yoga, a challenging traditional yoga practice.

Restorative Yoga for Life: A Relaxing Way to De-Stress, Re-Energize, and Find Balance by Gail Boorstein Grossman

Teaches restorative yoga poses and sequences to those who want to utilize yoga to relieve stress.

Yoga Anatomy by Leslie Kaminoff and Amy Matthews

An anatomy guide to help you improve your practice through a better understanding of basic anatomy.

Websites

beYogi
beyogi.com

Eckhart Yoga
ekhartyoga.com

Solstice Yoga
solsticeyoga.org

Yoga International
yogainternational.com

REFERENCES

Centers for Disease Control and Prevention. "Physical Inactivity." Accessed March 20, 2022. cdc.gov/chronicdisease/resources/publications/factsheets /physical-activity.htm.

Ghauri, Majid. "Does Physical Inactivity Lead to Chronic Pain?" Spine and Pain Clinics of North America. Last modified August 10, 2021. sapnamed.com/blog /does-physical-inactivity-lead-to-chronic-pain.

Harvard Health Publishing. "The Importance of Stretching." Harvard Medical School. Last modified March 14, 2022. health.harvard.edu/staying-healthy /the-importance-of-stretching#:~:text=Why%20stretching%20is%20important, muscles%20shorten%20and%20become%20tight.&text=That%20puts%20 you%20at%20risk,%2C%20strains%2C%20and%20muscle%20damage.

Harvard Health Publishing. "In a Slump? Fix Your Posture." Harvard Medical School. Accessed March 20, 2022. health.harvard.edu/staying-healthy/in-a -slump-fix-your-posture.

Kim, Si-Hyun, Oh-Yun Kwon, Kyue-Nam Park, In-Cheol Jeon, and Jong-Hyuck Weon. "Lower Extremity Strength and the Range of Motion in Relation to Squat Depth." *Journal of Human Kinetics* 45, no. 1 (2015): 59–69. doi.org/10.1515/hukin-2015-0007.

Law, Laura Frey, and Kathleen A. Sluka. "How Does Physical Activity Modulate Pain?" *Pain* 158, no. 3 (2017): 369–70. doi.org/10.1097/j.pain.0000000000000792.

Mayo Clinic. "Stretching: Focus on Flexibility." Last modified February 12, 2022. mayoclinic.org/healthy-lifestyle/fitness/in-depth/stretching/art-20047931.

Nassif, Thomas H., Deborah O. Norris, Karen L. Soltes, Marc R. Blackman, Julie C. Chapman, and Friedhelm Sandbrink. "Evaluating the Effectiveness of Mind-fulness Meditation for Chronic Musculoskeletal Pain in U.S. Veterans Using the Defense and Veterans Pain Rating Scale (DVPRS)." *Pain Medicine* 211, no. 15 (2014): 529–30.

Park, Juyoung, Cheryl A. Krause-Parello, and Chrisanne M. Barnes. "A Narrative Review of Movement-Based Mind-Body Interventions: Effects of Yoga, Tai Chi, and Qigong for Back Pain Patients." *Holistic Nursing Practice* 34, no. 1 (2020): 3–23. doi.org/10.1097/HNP.0000000000000360.

Polsgrove, M. Jay, Brandon M. Eggleston, and Roch J. Lockyer. "Impact of 10 Weeks of Yoga Practice on Flexibility and Balance of College Athletes." *International Journal of Yoga* 9, no. 1 (2016): 27–34. doi.org/10.4103/0973 -6131.171710.

Shohani, Masoumeh, Gholamreza Badfar, Marzieh Parizad Nasirkandy, et al. "The Effect of Yoga on Stress, Anxiety, and Depression in Women." *International Journal of Preventive Medicine* 9, no. 21 (2018). doi.org/10.4103 /ijpvm.IJPVM_242_16.

Tolahunase, Madhuri, Rajesh Sagar, and Rima Dada. "Impact of Yoga and Meditation on Cellular Aging in Apparently Healthy Individuals: A Prospective, Open-Label Single-Arm Exploratory Study." *Oxidative Medicine and Cellular Longevity* (2017): 7928981. doi.org/10.1155/2017/7928981.

INDEX

Acknowledgments

I have to start by thanking my amazing husband, Mike Gushue, who took charge of home renovations and held up the sky while I wrote this book.

Thanks to everyone on the Callisto team, especially Rachelle Cihonski, who patiently answered all my questions, no matter how many flooded her inbox.

I don't believe I'd ever get anything done without my sister and best friend, Karina. Thank you for co-working with me and for being my sounding board.

Finally, I'd like to thank my family for their unwavering support and their belief in me, especially my parents, Lourdes and Jim.

About the Author

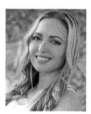 **Adriana Lee** is a Las Vegas–based yoga teacher, writer, content creator, and yoga teacher trainer. Known as @adrianainflow on Instagram and TikTok, she shares her knowledge and love of yoga on social media and as a regular contributing author for *beYogi*. Lee teaches at festivals nationally and online for Solstice Yoga as one of its co-owners. You can find her online at adrianainflow.com.